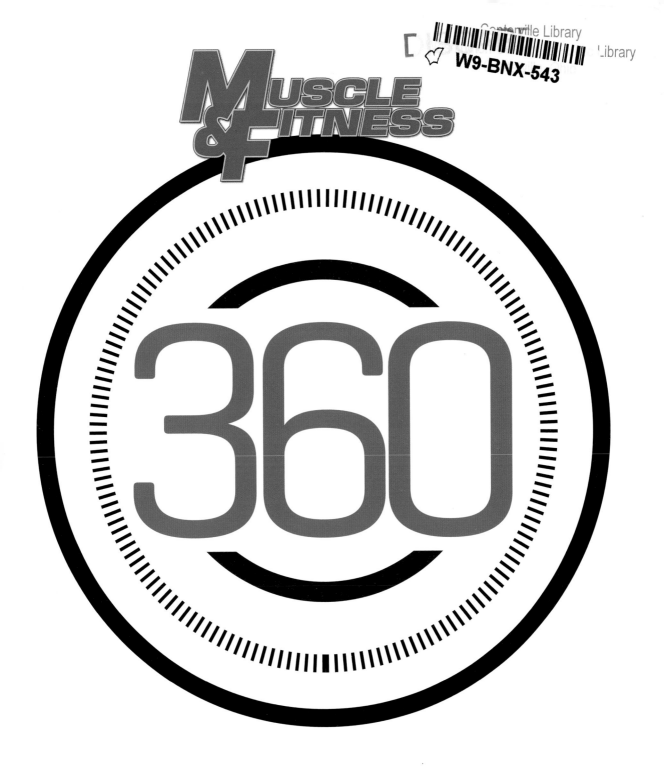

ACKNOWLEDGMENTS

This publication is based on articles written by **John Berardi, Ph.D.; Bob Bohnam; Jesse Burdick; Steve Cotter; Rob Fitzgerald; Sean Hyson; Matthew Kadey; John Meadows; CJ Murphy; Jimmy Pena; Jim Stoppani, Ph.D.; Mark Thorpe;** and **Joe Wuebben**

Cover photography by **Patrik Giardino**

Photography and illustrations by **Marius Bugge, Dylan Coulter, Michael Darter, Jason Ellis, JJ Miller, Matt Salacuse, Ian Spanier,** and **Pavel Ythjall**

Project editor is **Joe Wuebben**

Project creative director is **Anthony Scerri**

Project copy editor is **Cat Perry**

Project photo assistant is **Anthony Nolan**

Founding chairman is **Joe Weider.** Chairman and CEO of American Media, Inc., is **David Pecker.**

This book is available in quantity at special discounts for your group or organization. For further information, contact:

Triumph Books LLC
814 North Franklin Street
Chicago, IL 60610
(312) 337-0747
www.triumphbooks.com

ISBN: 978-1-60078-856-7

Printed in USA.

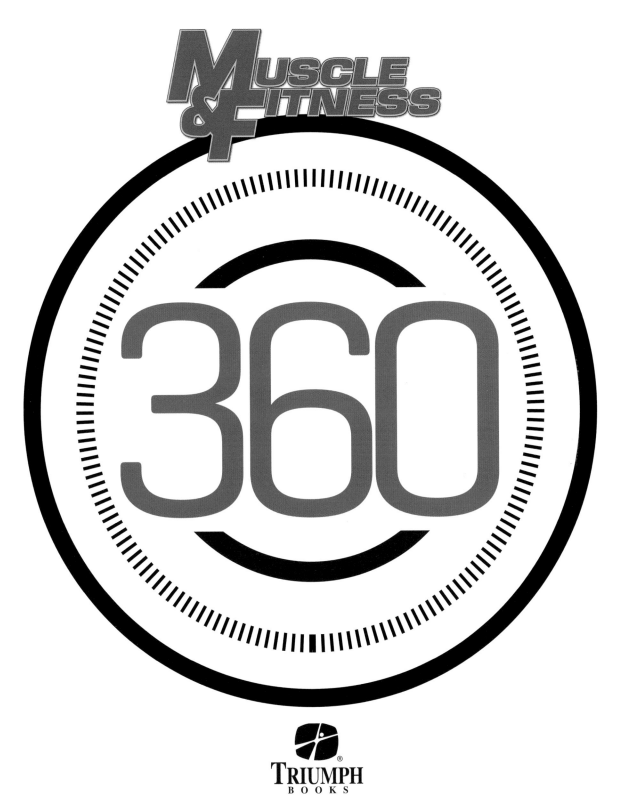

TRIUMPH
B O O K S

TRIUMPHBOOKS.COM

Contents

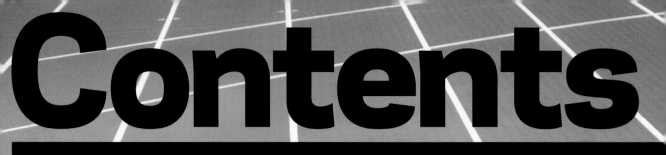

CHAPTER 1
ULTIMATE STARTER'S GUIDE
Never touched a weight before? Just coming back to the gym from a long hiatus? Either way, this comprehensive 8-week program is designed just for you.
PG 8

CHAPTER 2
TIME OUT FOR MUSCLE
Boost your size and strength—and burn more fat—by slashing your rest periods between sets.
PG 36

CHAPTER 3
DOUBLE YOUR GAINS
Two-a-day training pushes your muscles to the limit and speeds growth at a breakneck pace. Can you handle it?
PG 44

CHAPTER 4
BUILD BRUTE STRENGTH
Your body is your greatest project. We've got the blueprint to get you bigger and stronger than ever before.
PG 54

CHAPTER 5
UP THE INTENSITY
These seven intensity-boosting training techniques will push your workouts—and your physique—to the next level.
PG 64

CHAPTER 6
RAGE WITH THE MACHINES
Build muscle despite age or injuries with the right equipment.
PG 74

CHAPTER 7
ONE AND DONE
No matter what odd piece of equipment you have, we can make a hardcore workout with it.
PG 82

CHAPTER 8
RING THE BELL
Don't just get big. Build size, strength, and athletic power with Russia's greatest export: the kettlebell.
PG 92

CHAPTER 9
STEEL-BELTED STRENGTH
Drag your way to mass—and serious fat loss—with this inexpensive yet indispensable workout solution.
PG 100

CHAPTER 10
SPOT ON TRAINING
Attack your weak points, head to toe, with this physique troubleshooting guide.
PG 110

CHAPTER 11
THE NINE BEST EXERCISES YOU'RE NOT DOING
These muscle-building moves have been absent from your workouts for too long—maybe forever. It's time for a proper introduction.
PG 118

CHAPTER 12
SHOW-OFF MUSCLE
For a summer of T-shirts and shorts, build the three muscles they can see: your neck, forearms, and calves.
PG 126

CHAPTER 13
THE METABOLIC WORKOUT
Strip off excess body fat and take your conditioning to the next level with metabolic circuit training.
PG 134

CHAPTER 14
25 TIPS FOR MORE MUSCLE AND SUPER STRENGTH
Apply these concepts to outgrow your clothes and break your lifting records.
PG 142

CHAPTER 15
FAT-SEARING SEVEN
These track-inspired sprint programs will torch your fat while saving your muscle.
PG 154

CHAPTER 16
21 FOODS YOU SHOULD NEVER BE WITHOUT
If you want to build maximum muscle and torch body fat, make sure these foods are in your nutrition arsenal.
PG 164

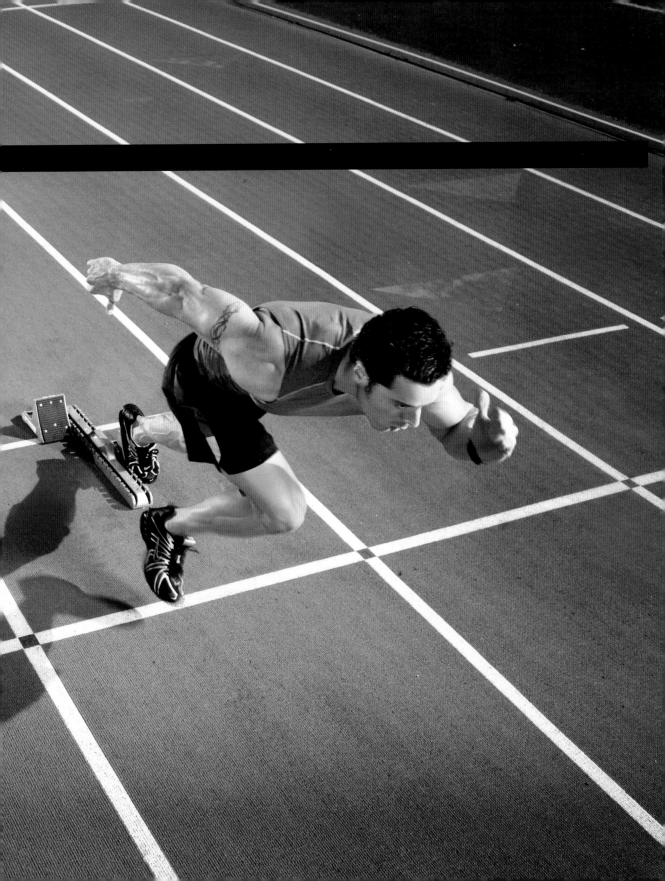

FOREWORD

LIFT YOUR WAY TO A STRONGER, HEALTHIER BODY

If you're like most Americans, you make sure to keep your car maintained and clean. You also keep an orderly home, brush your teeth every night, and get your hair cut when it starts to look unruly. You probably also mow your lawn, buy new clothes, and/or bring your pet to the vet for checkups regularly.

Yet, for all of our apparent diligence, a recent Centers for Disease Control and Prevention study has found that some 80% of Americans don't exercise enough to maintain optimal health. For all that we do take care of in our lives, the one thing we seem to neglect most is our bodies! Even worse, of those who do actually put in the CDC-recommended 2.5 hours of cardiovascular exercise or 1.5 hours of strength training per week, the vast majority opt for cardio only. Empirical evidence could have told me that, though. Whenever I'm at the gym I can't help but notice how much busier the cardio section is than the gym floor. In a way, I'm personally grateful for this—it makes working out easier when you've got the gym to yourself. However, the less selfish part of me wants to walk over to everyone crowding the recumbent bikes and treadmills and plead my case for the benefits of weight training.

Fact is, progressive resistance training—aka weight lifting or bodybuilding—is essential not just for those wishing to change their body composition, increase their biceps size, or get physically stronger. It can also strengthen bones and connective tissue, improve cognitive ability and circulation, and, if performed at a good pace, serve as a suitable substitute for traditional steady-state cardio like running and bicycling.

Not only is there a vast amount of clinical evidence for all of this, but I have my own personal evidence as well. You see, I don't do traditional cardio, ever. Yet I maintain under 7% body fat year-round without following a special fat-loss diet. I attribute my ability to stay so lean to my adherence to frequent, fast-paced workouts lasting around 75 minutes, five times per week. By keeping rest periods to under a minute—that means

not getting caught up in conversation or answering e-mails while on the gym floor—you too can reap all the rewards that progressive resistance training has to offer.

This book gives you a huge variety of options for training each of your major muscle groups. Some of the workouts may appeal more to you than others, but the only way you'll discover which you like most is to try as many as you can. Actually, there's clinical evidence that even that will benefit you: The body is a resilient, adaptive machine, designed to adjust to stresses placed upon it. By routinely switching up your workouts you will keep your body off-guard, thereby challenging it to always adapt to new stresses. If you were to stick with each routine in this book for the prescribed timeframe, for example, and then cycle to the next, you would be keeping your body guessing for at least the next couple of years!

Let me close by congratulating you on not being an 80-percenter. By virtue of the fact that you have this book in your hands, you are one of those who is already aware of the myriad benefits progressive resistance training has to offer, and someone who is motivated to be stronger, leaner, healthier, and physically better than ever before. We are, unfortunately, a minority in the United States, and dare I say, the world. But the more of us who follow the lead outlined in this book and by *Muscle & Fitness* magazine on a monthly basis, the more of us there are to help spread the word. Then maybe one day everyone will find themselves on the path to better health and vitality, just like you. But we can't help others until we help ourselves first, so here's to you. Salud!

More Power to You,
Shawn Perine
Editor-in-Chief, *Muscle & Fitness*

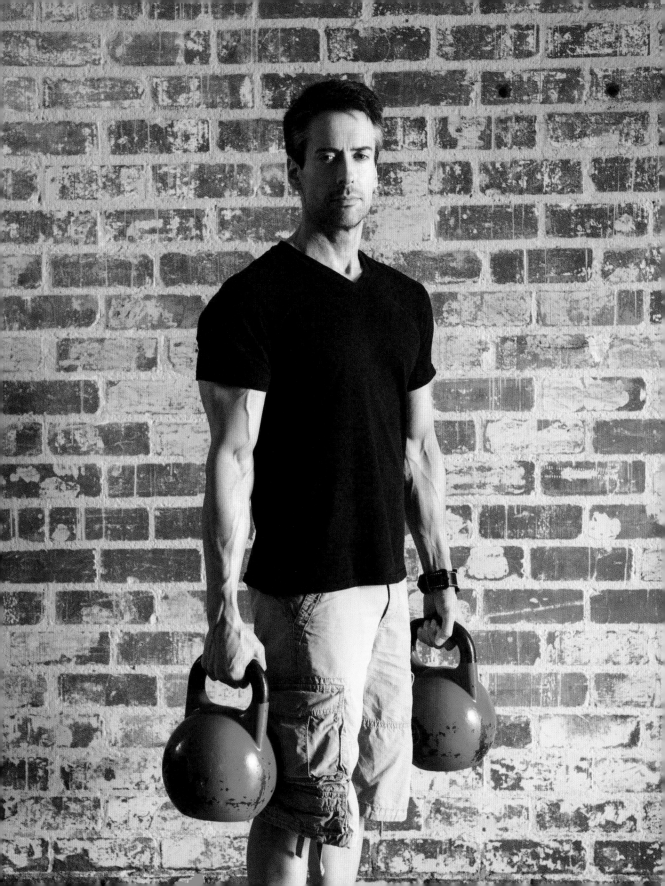

ULTIMATE STARTER'S GUIDE

The best athletes and bodybuilders in the world weren't born with superhuman strength and chiseled abs. At one point, they were just like you: a true newbie, a beginner, and not altogether certain of what to do first. In times like these, you need a blueprint to tell you exactly what to do in the gym, when to do it, and what kinds of foods and supplements to put in your body. That's what you have here in the very first chapter of this book—a starter's guide to get you going so that two months from now you'll be ready to graduate from beginner status with a bigger, stronger, leaner physique to show for it.

TRAINING - Pg. 10   **NUTRITION** - Pg. 26   **SUPPLEMENTS** - Pg. 32

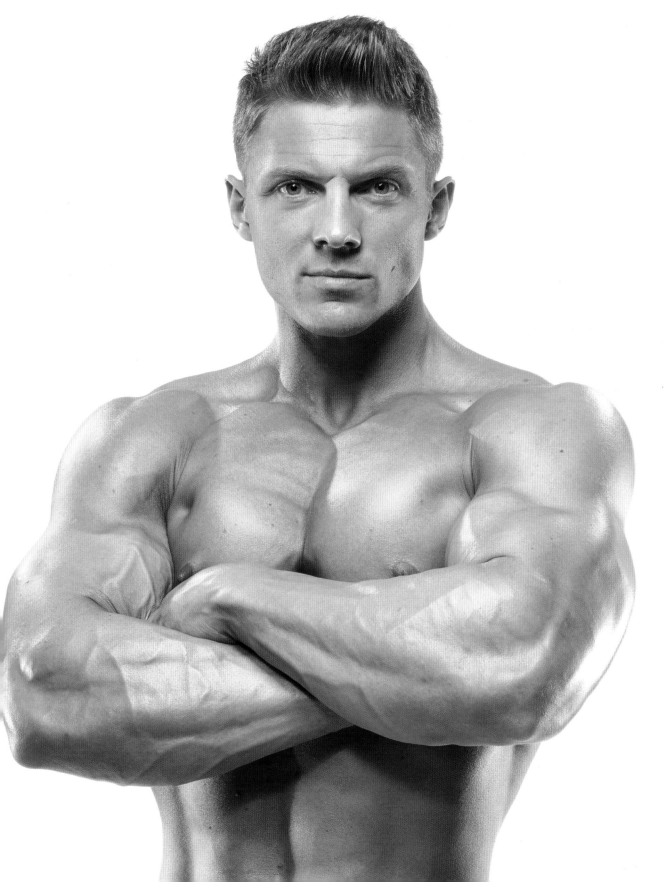

Training

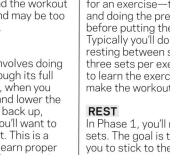

WHETHER you're a true beginner who's never had the pleasure of hoisting a loaded barbell overhead or you're simply getting back on the road to fitness after a long layoff, this is the perfect training plan to take you from novice to experienced lifter in just eight weeks. That's not to say that after two months you'll be ready to stand onstage next to reigning Mr. Olympia winner Phil Heath, but you will add considerable muscle mass and strength to your frame and set the table for more advanced training techniques you can try down the road.

This starter's program is grounded in progression—of the exercises you use, of the number of sets you complete per workout, in the amount of weight you use, and most important, in your training split. A training split is a system by which we divide up workouts according to muscle groups and days.

For example, some pro bodybuilders train only one major muscle group each workout. On Monday they may train chest, on Tuesday back, Wednesday legs, Thursday shoulders, and Friday arms (biceps and triceps), with abs thrown in one or two of those days for good measure. Since this splits up the body into five different workouts, it would be considered a five-day training split.

There's an infinite number of splits that can be devised, but specific splits exist that are more beneficial than others for developing a solid muscle base for the beginner. The example above would be too advanced for the newbie and would result in overtraining.

So what is the best training split for a beginner? One of the most effective is the whole-body split. (We'll get into the details of what that is in a minute.) The key is to continue using the proper split as you progress from beginner to advanced.

PHASE 1: WEEKS 1-2
(WHOLE-BODY TRAINING SPLIT)

As the name implies, a whole-body training split involves training your entire body in every workout. The major benefit of this for a beginner is that it allows you to train each muscle group more frequently—up to three times per week. This repetition is also important for training the body's nervous system.

Before you can focus on building serious muscle, you first need to train your muscles to contract properly. Learning how to bench-press or squat is like learning to ride a bike, just with less falling. Your muscle fibers need to learn how to contract synchronously so that you can perform the exercise correctly and apply the most strength when you do it. And the best way to learn how to do something is through repetition.

You'll be following a whole-body training split three times per week. We suggest training on Monday, Wednesday, and Friday, but any three days of the week will do, as long as you allow one day of rest from weight-training between workouts. Your body needs time to recover from the previous workout in order to make gains in muscle size and strength.

Phase 1 Rundown
EXERCISES

The exercises you will be using are tried-and-true mass builders that have been done for decades, if not centuries. These include exercises like the bench press, squat, and barbell curl, to name a few. You'll do one exercise per muscle group during this phase. Any more than that and the workout becomes prohibitively long and may be too much for uninitiated muscles.

REPS

A repetition ("rep," for short) involves doing a given exercise one time through its full range of motion. For example, when you lie down on the bench press and lower the bar to your chest and press it back up, that's one rep. In this phase you'll want to do around 10-12 reps per set. This is a good range for a beginner to learn proper exercise form and build muscle size and strength.

WEIGHT

The amount of weight you'll use is determined by the rep range. Since you'll be doing 10-12 reps per set, you should choose a weight that prevents you from doing any more than 12 reps but allows you to com- plete at least 10. Expect to get stronger over these three weeks, so once you can do more than 12 reps with the weight you're using, it's time to bump it up by 5-10 pounds.

SETS

A *set* is the term that refers to doing all r for an exercise—that is, picking up the ba and doing the prescribed number of reps before putting the bar down. That's one s Typically you'll do multiple sets per exerci resting between sets. In this phase, you'l three sets per exercise, which is just enou to learn the exercise yet not too much to make the workout drag on.

REST

In Phase 1, you'll rest 2-3 minutes betwe sets. The goal is to rest long enough to al you to stick to the rep range using the sa weight on all three sets. Research publish in the *Journal of Strength and Conditioni Research* has reported that beginner lifte resting 2½ minutes between sets gained more than twice as much muscle on their arms as those resting for one minute.

BENTOVER BARBELL ROW

Stand holding a barbell with a shoulder-width, overhand grip. Bend your knees slightly and bend over at your waist so your torso is close to parallel with the floor, maintaining this position throughout. Start with your arms hanging straight down, then pull the bar to your stomach, just below your rib cage. At the top of the move, squeeze your shoulder blades together to fully contract your back muscles, then slowly return the bar to the start position.

Phase 1 Workouts (WHOLE-BODY TRAINING SPLIT)

Do this workout three times per week with at least one day of rest between workouts (e.g., Monday, Wednesday, and Friday).

MUSCLE GROUP	EXERCISE	SETS/REPS	REST
Chest	Barbell Bench Press	3/10-12	2-3 min.
Back	Bentover Barbell Row	3/10-12	2-3 min.
Legs	Squat	3/10-12	2-3 min.
Shoulders	Barbell Shoulder Press	3/10-12	2-3 min.
Triceps	Triceps Pressdown	3/10-12	2-3 min.
Biceps	Barbell Curl	3/10-12	2-3 min.
Calves	Standing Calf Raise	3/12-15	1-2 min.
Abs	Crunch	3/To failure	1-2 min.

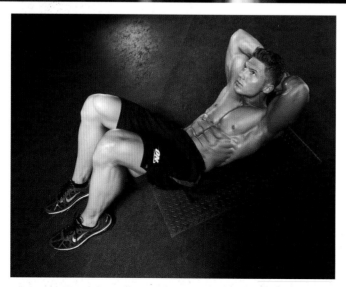

CRUNCH
Lie faceup on the floor with your knees bent 90 degrees and your feet flat on the floor. Position your arms either across your chest or with your hands behind your head. Contract your abs to lift your shoulder blades off the floor approximately six inches. Squeeze your abs for a count, then lower yourself slowly back to the floor. The range of motion on the crunch is very short—the goal is to press your lower back into the floor to bring your sternum closer to your pelvis.

BARBELL CURL

Stand holding a barbell with a shoulder-width grip, your arms extended toward the floor and your knees slightly bent. Keeping your torso erect (don't lean back while lifting the weight), contract your biceps to curl the weight up. Make sure your elbows remain at your sides throughout—don't let them flare out or lift up. Slowly lower the weight to the start position.

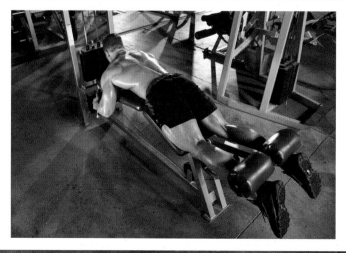

LYING LEG CURL
Adjust the machine so the roller pad sits on the backs of your ankles. Assume a prone position on the bench and stabilize yourself by grasping the handles. Start with your legs straight and the weight lifted a few inches off the stack. Flex your knees to curl the pad up toward your glutes. When the pad reaches your glutes, squeeze your hamstrings for a count, then slowly lower to the start position.

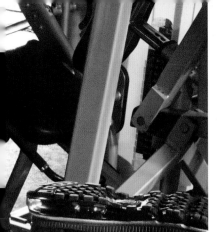

PHASE 2: WEEKS 3–4
(TWO-DAY TRAINING SPLIT)

After two weeks of following a whole-body split, it's time to give your muscles a new challenge. For the third and fourth weeks you'll move to a two-day training split repeated twice a week for a total of four weekly workouts. A two-day split means you'll divide up your entire body into two separate workouts, training half the body in one and the other half in the other. In this particular two-day split you'll train all your torso muscle groups (chest, back, shoulders, and abs) in Workout 1 and all your limb muscles (biceps, triceps, legs, and calves) in Workout 2.

One major benefit of moving up to a two-day training split is that it allows you to do more exercises per muscle group and to train each muscle group with more intensity. These are two critical components to making continued progress in the gym. To keep growing, muscles need to gradually do more work at higher intensity. Training fewer muscle groups per workout allows you to put more effort into those you're training by going heavier and making sure you take each set to muscle failure.

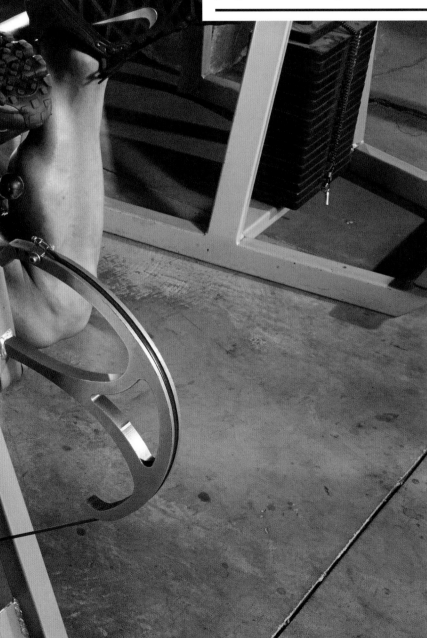

Phase 2 Rundown
EXERCISES

The exercises you'll be using here will be the major mass builders you started in Phase 1, plus some additional moves. For most muscle groups, this will allow you to do one multijoint mass builder and one single-joint (isolation) exercise to build both overall size and shape. You'll also add an exercise to work the trapezius, or traps, in this phase.

WEIGHT

You'll be going heavier this phase, at least on the first exercise for each muscle group. Find a weight that limits you to 8–10 reps on the first exercise and one that allows you to complete 10–12 reps on the second and third exercises. Again, once you can do more than the rep range listed for each exercise add 5–10 pounds, or whatever weight brings your reps into the listed rep range.

REPS

In Phase 2, you'll drop reps down to 8–10 per set on the first exercise for each muscle group. This allows you to train a bit heavier than the previous phase, which will help you build more strength and size. On the second and third exercises you'll keep the reps higher, at 10–12. Calves are an exception, and you'll need to increase the reps to 15–20.

REST

During this phase you'll rest about 2–3 minutes between sets to allow you to stick with heavier weight and complete more reps for maximizing strength and size gains.

SETS

You'll still be doing three sets per exercise; however, since you're now doing two exercises per muscle group (and three for legs), that's a jump in total sets per muscle group from three to six (or nine sets for legs). This increase in the amount of work you do for each muscle group is important for continued progress.

DUMBBELL SHRUG
Hold two dumbbells at arm's length next to your thighs. Keeping your elbows extended, simply elevate (or "shrug") your shoulders as high as you can—straight up and down, not backward or forward—and squeeze at the top. Return to the start position, depressing your shoulders. Repeat for reps.

CLINE DUMBBELL CURL

ust an incline bench to about 45-60 degrees
 sit back squarely against the bench, feet
 on the floor. Your arms should hang straight
vn by your sides, palms up. Keeping your
ulders back and upper arms in a fixed position
pendicular to the floor, curl the weights up so
 dumbbells approach your shoulders. Squeeze
r biceps hard at the top before slowly return-
back to the start position.

Phase 2 Workouts (TWO-DAY TRAINING SPLIT)

Do each of the following workouts twice per week. For example, do Workout 1 on Monday and then again on Thursday, and do Workout 2 on Tuesday and Friday.

WORKOUT 1

MUSCLE GROUP	EXERCISE	SETS/REPS	REST
Chest	Bench Press	3/8-10	2-3 min.
	Incline Dumbbell Flye	3/10-12	2-3 min.
Back	Barbell Bentover Row	3/8-10	2-3 min.
	Lat Pulldown	3/10-12	2-3 min.
Shoulders	Barbell Shoulder Press	3/8-10	2-3 min.
	Dumbbell Lateral Raise	3/10-12	2-3 min.
Traps	Barbell Shrug	3/8-10	2-3 min.
Abdominals	Reverse Crunch	3/To failure	1-2 min.
	Crunch	3/To failure	1-2 min.

WORKOUT 2

MUSCLE GROUP	EXERCISE	SETS/REPS	REST
Biceps	Barbell Curl	3/8-10	2-3 min.
	Incline Dumbbell Curl	3/10-12	2-3 min.
Triceps	Close-grip Bench Press	3/8-10	2-3 min.
	Triceps Pressdown	3/10-12	2-3 min.
Legs	Squat	3/8-10	2-3 min.
	Leg Extension	3/10-12	2-3 min.
	Lying Leg Curl	3/10-12	2-3 min.
Calves	Standing Calf Raise	2/15-20	1-2 min.
	Seated Calf Raise	2/15-20	1-2 min.

PHASE 3: WEEKS 5-6
(THREE-DAY TRAINING SPLIT)

With four weeks of consistent training under your belt you should be very comfortable with your form on the exercises you've been doing, as your nervous system and muscle fibers are getting properly trained through the constant repetition. In Week 5, it's time to step up both the amount of work you're doing for each muscle group and the intensity yet again. Remember, the goal here is to keep progressing, and the only way to do that is to keep raising the bar.

Phase 3 progresses to a three-day training split, where, instead of dividing the body up into two different workouts, you'll be dividing it three ways. This means you'll train fewer muscle groups each workout, which allows you to do more exercises per muscle group and train each muscle group with even greater intensity.

Although there are numerous ways to pair muscle groups to work with a three-day split, one of the most effective is known as a push/pull/legs split. That means the body is broken down into a push day, where you train all the pushing muscles of the upper body (chest, shoulders, and triceps); a pull day, where you train all the pulling muscles of the upper body (back, traps, biceps, and forearms); and a leg day (legs and calves).

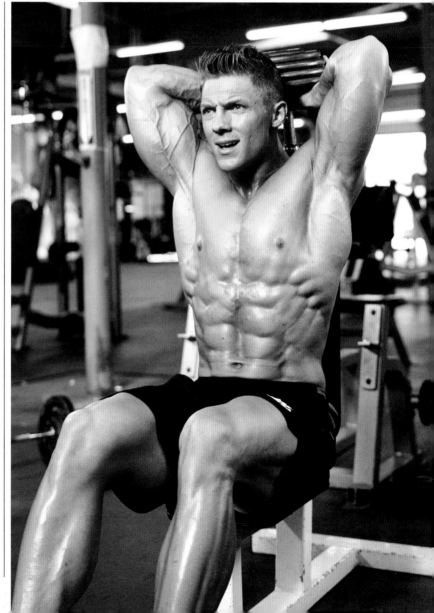

DUMBBELL OVERHEAD TRICEPS EXTENSIO
Sit on a low-back seat with your feet flat on th floor. Grasp the inner plate of a dumbbell with both hands and hold it overhead with your elbo extended. Bending only at your elbows, lower the weight behind your head until you feel a de stretch in your triceps. Extend your elbows an squeeze your triceps at the top.

Phase 3 Rundown
EXERCISES

This phase contains the same exercises as the previous phases, with an additional exercise added to most muscle groups; to build well-developed muscles, you need to target different areas of them. You'll also add an exercise for a new group: forearms.

WEIGHT

As you've been doing in Phases 1 and 2, choose the proper weight that allows you to hit the listed rep range for each exercise. And continue to add weight when you find yourself able to compete more reps than the listed rep range.

REPS

Excluding calves, abs, and forearms, you'll drop down to 6-8 reps per set for your first exercise per muscle group. The second exercise will be 8-10 reps, and the last exercise will be 12-15 reps.

REST

During this phase you'll also rest about 2-3 minutes between sets to allow you to stick with heavier weight and complete more reps for maximizing strength and size gains.

SETS

You'll still be doing three sets per exercise. However, since you're now adding another exercise for most muscle groups, you'll be doing an extra three sets per muscle group.

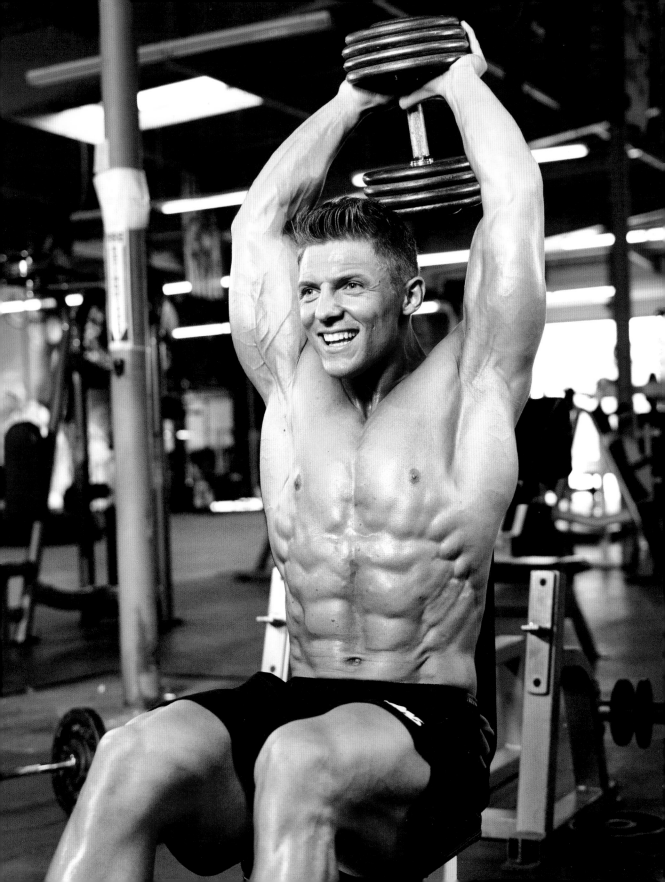

Phase 3 Workouts (THREE-DAY TRAINING SPLIT)

Do each workout once a week, allowing at least one day of rest between workouts.

WORKOUT 1
PUSH DAY

MUSCLE GROUP	EXERCISE	SETS/REPS	REST
Chest	Bench Press	3/6-8	2-3 min.
	Incline Dumbbell Bench Press	3/8-10	2-3 min.
	Incline Dumbbell Flye	3/12-15	2-3 min.
Shoulders	Barbell Shoulder Press	3/6-8	2-3 min.
	Smith Machine Upright Row	3/8-10	2-3 min.
	Dumbbell Lateral Raise	3/12-15	2-3 min.
Triceps	Close-grip Bench Press	3/6-8	2-3 min.
	Dumbbell Overhead Triceps Extension	3/8-10	2-3 min.
	Triceps Pressdown	3/12-15	2-3 min.

WORKOUT 2
LEG DAY

MUSCLE GROUP	EXERCISE	SETS/REPS	REST
Legs	Squat	3/6-8	2-3 min.
	Leg Press	3/8-10	2-3 min.
	Leg Extension	3/12-15	2-3 min.
	Lying Leg Curl	3/12-15	2-3 min.
Calves	Standing Calf Raise	3/20-25	1-2 min.
	Seated Calf Raise	3/20-25	1-2 min.
Abdominals	Reverse Crunch	3/To failure	1-2 min.
	Crunch	3/To failure	1-2 min.
	Oblique Cable Crunch	3/To failure	1-2 min.

WORKOUT 3
PULL DAY

MUSCLE GROUP	EXERCISE	SETS/REPS	REST
Back	Bentover Barbell Row	3/6-8	2-3 min.
	Lat Pulldown	3/8-10	2-3 min.
	Seated Cable Row	3/12-15	2-3 min.
Traps	Barbell Shrug	3/6-8	2-3 min.
Biceps	Barbell Curl	3/6-8	2-3 min.
	Incline Dumbbell Curl	3/8-10	2-3 min.
	Preacher Curl	3/12-15	2-3 min.
Forearms	Wrist Curl	3/10-12	1-2 min.

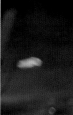

INCLINE DUMBBELL BENCH PRESS
Lie faceup on an incline bench with your feet flat on the floor. Hold a dumbbell in each hand just outside your shoulders. Powerfully press the dumbbells upward toward the ceiling, stopping when the dumbbells are an inch or so away from each other, then slowly return the dumbbells to the start and repeat.

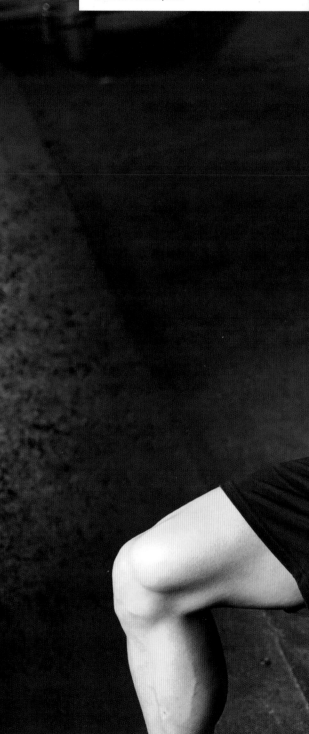

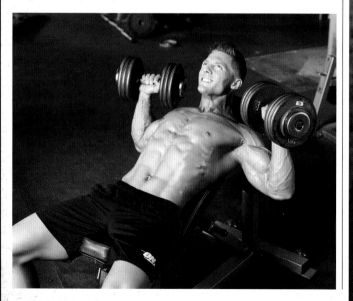

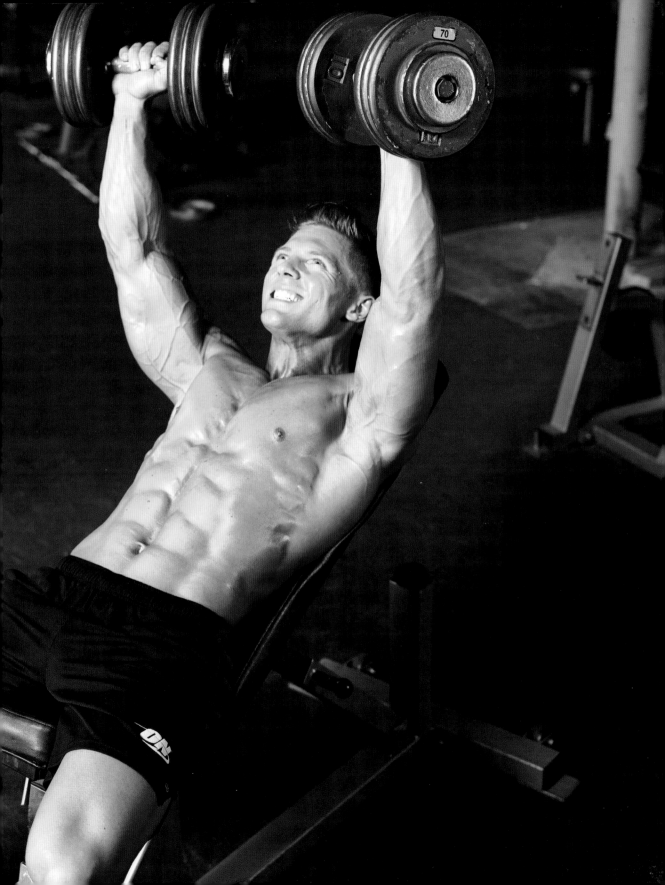

CABLE CROSSOVER
Stand in the middle of a two-sided cable station with D-handles attached to both high-pulley cables. Begin with your arms extended out to your sides and elbows slightly bent. Step forward to make sure the weights aren't resting on the stacks, then contract your pecs to pull your hands together, maintaining the slight bend in your elbows. At the end of the motion, cross your hands and squeeze your pecs for a count.

PHASE 4: WEEKS 7-8
(FOUR-DAY TRAINING SPLIT)

After six weeks of consistent training, you're in the home stretch of graduating from "starter" status. By now you should be realizing significant gains in muscle strength as well as mass and definition. This final phase completes your transition and will prepare you to train among intermediate and advanced lifters.

Now you'll be training your entire body over the course of four workouts. This will help you further increase the amount of work you can do for each muscle group and the intensity you can put into training each. This four-day split divides your body into the following workouts: chest, triceps, and abs; back, biceps, and forearms; legs and calves; and shoulders, traps, and abs. (You'll be training abs twice a week now. Because they're postural muscles that help with maintaining your upright posture all day, the abs can withstand more frequent training and actually respond well to it.)

Once you've completed this final phase, you'll be ready to take on advanced, high-intensity training techniques like supersets, dropsets, rest-pause, and extended sets, to name a few.

MANIAN DEADLIFT

nd upright holding a barbell in front of your up-thighs with an alternating grip (shown above). p your feet shoulder-width apart and have a t bend in your knees. Keeping your chest up, tight, and the natural arch in your lower back, n your hips back until your torso is roughly llel to the floor. Slide the bar down your thighs it reaches your shins. Extend your hips to g the bar back to the start position.

Phase 4 Rundown
EXERCISES

Another exercise has been added to most groups. Triceps and biceps will not need an additional exercise added, since these smaller muscle groups generally require less total work than larger muscle groups like chest, back, shoulders, and legs. The progress in the biceps and triceps will come from the weight and rep ranges used.

REPS

The exercise you do first for each major muscle group (excluding calves, abs, and forearms) will drop down to 4–6 reps per set to maximize strength gains. The second exercise will entail 6–8 reps per set for building strength and size. The last exercise or two will jump to 15–20 reps per set. Research from Japan has shown that combining heavy weight and lower reps with lighter weight sets for higher reps enhances both strength and muscle mass gains.

WEIGHT

Again, choose a weight for each exercise that allows you to hit the listed rep range. Continue to increase the weight as you can complete more reps than the prescribed rep range.

REST

During this phase you'll rest 2–3 minutes between sets when you're using heavier weight and low reps. However, you'll now drop rest periods between sets to just one minute on lighter-weight sets where higher reps are performed. This will help maximize growth hormone levels, which will lead to further gains in muscle size and strength as well encourage fat loss for greater definition.

SETS

You'll still be doing three sets per exercise, but the added exercises will increase the total number of sets performed.

Phase 4 Workouts (FOUR-DAY TRAINING SPLIT)

Do each workout below once per week, such as Workout 1 on Monday, Workout 2 on Tuesday, Workout 3 on Thursday, and Workout 4 on Friday.

WORKOUT 1

MUSCLE GROUP	EXERCISE	SETS/REPS	REST
Chest	Bench Press	3/4-6	2-3 min.
	Dumbbell Incline Bench Press	3/6-8	2-3 min.
	Incline Dumbbell Flye	3/15-20	1 min.
	Cable Crossover	3/15-20	1 min.
Triceps	Close-grip Bench Press	3/4-6	2-3 min.
	Dumbbell Overhead Triceps Extension	3/6-8	2-3 min.
	Triceps Pressdown	3/15-20	1 min.
Abdominals	Hanging Leg Raise	3/To failure	1 min.
	Double Crunch	3/To failure	1 min.
	Plank	3/1 min.	1 min.

WORKOUT 2

MUSCLE GROUP	EXERCISE	SETS/REPS	REST
Back	Barbell Row	3/4-6	2-3 min.
	Lat Pulldown	3/6-8	2-3 min.
	Seated Cable Row	3/15-20	1 min.
	Straight-arm Pulldown	3/15-20	1 min.
Biceps	Barbell Curl	3/4-6	2-3 min.
	Incline Dumbbell Curl	3/6-8	2-3 min.
	Preacher Curl	3/15-20	1 min.
Forearms	Wrist Curl	3/12-15	1 min.
	Reverse-grip Wrist Curl	3/12-15	1 min.

WORKOUT 3

MUSCLE GROUP	EXERCISE	SETS/REPS	REST
Legs	Squat	3/4-6	2-3 min.
	Leg Press	3/4-6	2-3 min.
	Leg Extension	3/15-20	1 min.
	Romanian Deadlift	3/4-6	2-3 min.
	Lying Leg Curl	3/15-20	1 min.
Calves	Standing Calf Raise	3/25-30	1 min.
	Seated Calf Raise	3/25-30	1 min.

WORKOUT 4

MUSCLE GROUP	EXERCISE	SETS/REPS	REST
Shoulders	Barbell Shoulder Press	3/4-6	2-3 min.
	Smith Machine Upright Row	3/6-8	2-3 min.
	Dumbbell Lateral Raise	3/15-20	1 min.
	Dumbbell Rear-delt Raise	3/15-20	1 min.
Traps	Barbell Shrug	3/4-6	2-3 min.
	Dumbbell Shrug	3/15-20	1 min.
Abdominals	Reverse Crunch	3/To failure	1 min.
	Crunch	3/To failure	1 min.
	Oblique Cable Crunch	3/15-20	1 min.

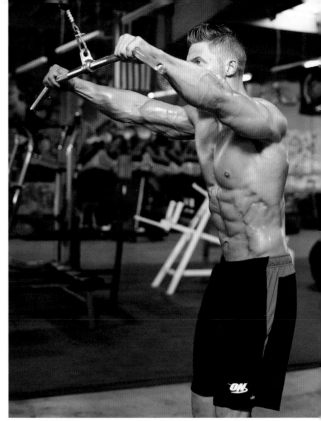

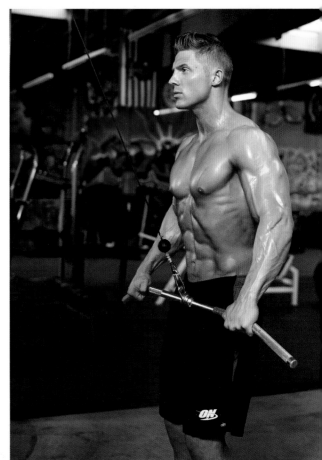

STRAIGHT-ARM PULLDOWN

Stand facing a cable stack and attach a straight bar or rope handle to a high-pulley cable. Grasp the attachment with both hands and begin with your arms extended in front of you roughly at head height. (Make sure the weight isn't resting on the stack.) Contract your lats to pull the weight down toward your thighs, keeping your elbows extended to isolate your back muscles.

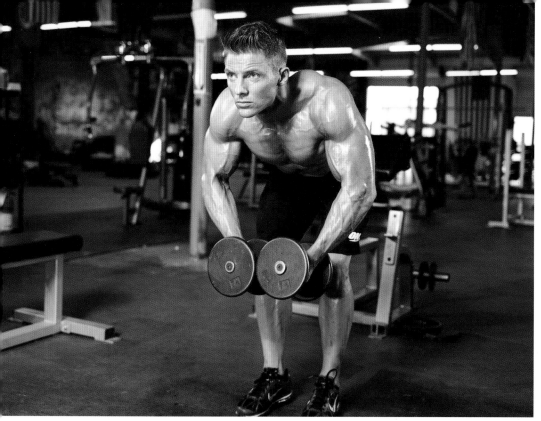

DUMBBELL REAR-DELT RAISE

Hold a pair of dumbbells and stand with your feet shoulder-width apart. Bend at the waist until your upper body is almost parallel to the floor. Keep your back flat and raise the weights out to your sides as high as you can, keeping your elbows extended. Squeeze your rear delts at the top of the movement, and hold the weights there for a second. Slowly lower them back to the start position, and don't use momentum; start the next rep from a dead stop.

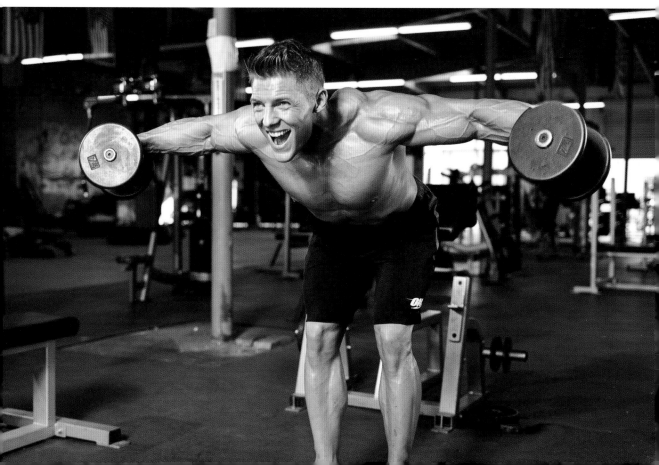

Nutrition

WHAT you do in the gym is only part of the equation for building a better body. What you eat, how much, and when, is just as significant to the development of a great physique, to both newbies and finely tuned athletes alike. Nutrition can be an overwhelming topic, evidenced by the abundance of diet books available today. To simplify things, we boiled it down to the 10 most critical "rules" of nutrition that, when followed, will provide you with the fuel you need for the body you want. Most beginners entering the weight room for the first time are looking to build muscle size and strength, which is why our rules focus on mass building first and foremost. But if you're a beginner who wants to lose some body fat while building muscle, then these same rules still apply, only with a few simple tweaks, as presented in the "Get-Lean Guidelines" in the text.

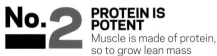

No.1 CALORIES COUNT

The first thing you need to focus on is consuming adequate calories. Building muscle is a calorie-intensive process. If you're not getting enough calories for daily bodily processes and repair, your body won't expend energy on muscle growth. On workout days, most guys will need about 18 calories per pound of body weight just to maintain their muscle mass. To increase that mass, you'll want to shoot for around 20–22 calories per pound, which equates to 3,000–3,300 calories for the 150-pound guy. On rest days, since you won't be expending as many calories, you can pull back your calorie intake to about 18 calories per pound (2,700 calories for the 150-pounder); this is mainly achieved by not consuming your pre- and post-workout meals. This will help to keep your mass gain on the lean side and avoid storing fat.
*Get-Lean Guideline: For those needing to lose fat, keep calories down at around 18 per pound of body weight on workout days and about 14–16 on rest days.

No.2 PROTEIN IS POTENT

Muscle is made of protein, so to grow lean mass you need to eat protein. Ample protein. Research now confirms that those who train with weights need at least 1 gram of protein per pound of body weight per day to build adequate muscle. And several studies show that bumping protein up to 1.5 grams per pound is very effective for gaining muscle when you're following a weight-training program. This is especially true when a good portion of that extra protein comes from whey.

At M&F, we've seen major gains in lean muscle mass in thousands and thousands of guys when they bump their protein up to 1.5 grams per pound on rest days and 2 grams per pound on workout days, even consuming as much as 40% of calories from protein. For the 150-pound guy that means consuming 225–300 grams of protein per day. As far as sources go, you need plenty of whey and casein protein (for more on whey and casein protein, see the starter's supplement section), but also lots of whole-food protein sources like eggs, lean beef, chicken, fish, and dairy.

No.3 CARBS ARE CRITICAL TOO

While carbohydrates may not be as critical as protein for muscle growth, they're still of vital importance. As we've discussed, your body needs to know it has an energy surplus to grow muscle most effectively. One signal your body uses to determine your energy status is through glycogen, the storage form of carbs in muscles and the liver. Glycogen pulls water into the muscle; the more glycogen you have stored in your muscles, the more water it pulls in, making your muscles fuller. This, in turn, places a stretch on the cell membranes, which instigates processes that increase muscle protein synthesis and can lead to long-term growth. On workout days you should be shooting for a minimum of around 2 grams of carbs per pound of body weight. That's at least 300 grams for a 150-pound person. On rest days, to keep fat gains at bay, drop carbs down to about 1.5 grams per pound; foregoing pre- and post-workout meals (because you're not working out) should account for this decrease in carbs.
*Get-Lean Guideline: For those needing to drop body fat, limit carbs to just 1 gram per pound of body weight per day on workout days and as low as 0.5 grams on rest days.

No.4 DON'T FORGET THE FAT

Fat is not the demon it was once thought to be. Men need a good amount of fat, even saturated fat, to maximize natural levels of testosterone. Monounsaturated fat is also critical for maintaining testosterone levels as well as enhancing overall health. And the essential omega-3 fats, such as

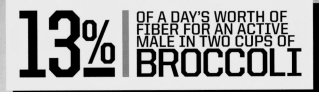

13% OF A DAY'S WORTH OF FIBER FOR AN ACTIVE MALE IN TWO CUPS OF **BROCCOLI**

those found in salmon and other fatty fish, encourage better muscle growth and joint recovery, not to mention all the health benefits it offers. You should shoot for at least half of your body weight in grams of fat. That's at least 75 grams of fat per day for the 150-pound guy. About ⅓ of that should be saturated fat, another ⅓ monounsaturated fat, and the other ⅓ polyunsaturated fat, with emphasis on omega-3 polyunsaturated fats.

No.5 EAT FREQUENTLY

We've long recommended frequent meals throughout the day for building muscle. Our sample meal plan (starting later in this chapter) is composed of seven meals on rest days and up to nine meals on workout days, with most meals spaced 2–3 hours apart. This strategy works well for building muscle, as we've seen in hundreds of thousands of guys, if not millions, over the years. This is also how we've evolved to eat as infants when our whole purpose in life is to increase mass as rapidly as possible.

One new study supports this concept. Researchers in Australia had subjects perform a leg workout and then fed them a total of 80 grams of whey protein over the next 12 hours in three different methods—either by consuming eight 10-gram doses every 1.5 hours; four 20-gram doses every three hours; or two 40-gram doses every six hours. They reported in a 2012 issue of the journal *Nutrition & Metabolism* that protein retention (the amount of protein retained from the whey in the muscle fibers) increased significantly more when subjects consumed the four 20-gram doses every three hours. The take-home point here: Consume a minimum of 20 grams of protein per meal and don't go any longer than three hours between meals to maximize muscle growth.

No.6 BREAK THE FAST

The 6–8-hour fast while you sleep signals your body to break down muscle protein for fuel, which is the last thing you want when trying to build muscle. Your body is very protective of the brain and central nervous system, which run on glucose (carbs). When you sleep, the majority of that glucose is supplied by the liver, which stocks up on stored carbs in the form of glycogen. When the glycogen levels of the liver reach a certain low point during the night, the liver signals the body to break down more muscle protein to convert the amino acids into glucose.

The first thing you should do when you wake up is stop this process by delivering a quick dose of branched-chain amino acids (BCAAs) and whey. You also want to restock liver glycogen. For this, we recommend fruit. Most fruit is low glycemic and made up of half or more fructose, so it doesn't flood your bloodstream with glucose; rather, it takes a direct trip to the liver where it is converted to glycogen and is slowly released as glucose. Eat a piece of fruit with 20 grams of whey and 5 grams of BCAAs to restock the liver and stop muscle protein breakdown. About 30–60 minutes later, eat a second breakfast of whole foods like eggs and oatmeal.

No.7

BE AN EGGHEAD

When it comes to protein, there are certain ones you should try to include in your diet on most days, if not every day. For starters, there's dairy protein, as discussed above. But another one that you should highly consider is eggs. We suggest you eat at least three whole eggs per day. Research has shown that men who eat three egg yolks daily while weight training gain twice as much muscle mass and strength as those not eating the yolks. This is likely due to the saturated fat and cholesterol in eggs aiding testosterone production. If you're worried about the cholesterol, don't. Research from the University of Connecticut shows that the cholesterol from egg yolks won't raise levels of bad cholesterol (LDL).

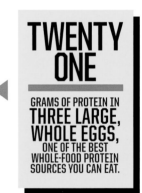

TWENTY ONE

GRAMS OF PROTEIN IN **THREE LARGE, WHOLE EGGS,** ONE OF THE BEST WHOLE-FOOD PROTEIN SOURCES YOU CAN EAT.

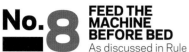

No.8 FEED THE MACHINE BEFORE BED

As discussed in Rule No. 6, you need to minimize the amount of muscle-protein breakdown that occurs while you sleep. Some bodybuilders have been so adamant about stopping this process that they actually set an alarm to wake up in the middle of the night and eat. Rest assured, you shouldn't need to go to such extremes if you prep before bed properly. Slow-digesting protein is your friend here. Anything that's rich in the milk-protein casein will provide a steady supply of amino acids for up to seven hours while you sleep, as casein is a very slow-digesting protein that provides your body a steady stream of aminos to help keep muscles intact. Good sources of casein include casein and milk protein powders, cottage cheese, Greek yogurt, and regular cheese such as string, American, and cheddar. Immediately before you go to bed, have one or two scoops of a casein-rich protein powder, a cup or so of cottage cheese or Greek yogurt, or 3–4 ounces of cheese.

No.9 BEEF UP

Another source of protein you'll want to be sure to eat is beef. In addition to the quality protein it provides, the saturated fat and cholesterol will enhance testosterone levels for maximizing muscle growth. Plus, beef is rich in B vitamins, zinc, and iron, all of which are critical for growing muscle and maintaining energy levels during workouts. They'll also help to keep your immune system strong, fighting off colds and other viruses that may force you to skip workouts and lose muscle.

No.10 EAT YOUR VEGGIES

When it comes to building muscle, a mistake that many make is to focus solely on macronutrients (protein, carbs, and fat). Yes, these should be high on your priority list, but you don't want to miss out on beneficial micronutrients (vitamins and minerals) and phytochemicals that vegetables are rich sources of. Not only do these micronutrients help to promote better overall health, but they can also help your body produce more testosterone, growth hormone, and nitric oxide (NO) to better promote gains in lean muscle.

SAMPLE DAILY DIETS

How to best plan your meals throughout the day depends partly on when you workout. The following four sample meal plans map out exactly what and when to eat based on your training schedule.

For those training in the evening (around 6 p.m.)…

BREAKFAST 1
- **½** cantaloupe
- **1 scoop** whey protein
- **5g** BCAAs

BREAKFAST 2
- **3** whole eggs
- **3** egg whites
- **2 cups** cooked oatmeal
- **1 tbsp** honey (add to oatmeal to sweeten)

LATE MORNING SNACK
- **1 cup** reduced-fat Greek yogurt
- **½** scoop whey protein (your favorite flavor)
- **1 tsp** honey
- **½ oz** walnuts (7 halves), crushed
(Mix all ingredients in Greek yogurt and enjoy.)

LUNCH
- **5 oz** can tuna (in water)
- **1 tbsp** light mayonnaise
- **2** slices whole-wheat bread (or Ezekiel bread)

MIDDAY SNACK
- **3** sticks light mozzarella string cheese
- **1** large whole-wheat pita bread
- **¼ cup** hummus
(Slice pita into triangles and dip in hummus.)

PRE-WORKOUT
- **1** large apple
- **1** scoop whey protein
- **5g** BCAAs
- **1** dose creatine

WORKOUT

POST-WORKOUT
- **1** scoop whey protein
- **2 cups** low-fat milk
- **10** Wonka Pixy Stix
- **5g** BCAAs
- **1** dose creatine

DINNER
- **8 oz** top sirloin steak
- **1** large sweet potato
- **2 cups** mixed green salad
- **2 tbsp** olive oil and vinegar-based dressing

BEDTIME SNACK
- **2 cups** popcorn
- **1 cup** low-fat cottage cheese

Daily Totals: 3,333 calories, 300g protein, 335g carbs, 85g fat

For those training in the morning…

BREAKFAST
1/Pre-workout

- **½** cantaloupe
- **1** scoop whey protein
- **5g** BCAAs
- **1** dose creatine

WORKOUT

POST-WORKOUT
- **1** scoop whey protein
- **2 cups** low-fat milk
- **10** Wonka Pixy Stix
- **5g** BCAAs
- **1** dose creatine

BREAKFAST 2
- **3** whole eggs
- **3** egg whites
- **2 cups** cooked oatmeal
- **1 tbsp** honey (add to oatmeal to sweeten)

LATE-MORNING SNACK
- **1 cup** reduced-fat Greek yogurt
- **½** scoop whey protein (your favorite flavor)
- **1 tsp** honey
- **½ oz** walnuts (7 halves), crushed
(Mix all ingredients in Greek yogurt and enjoy.)

LUNCH
- **5 oz** can tuna (in water)
- **1 tbsp** light mayonnaise
- **2** slices whole-wheat bread (or Ezekiel bread)

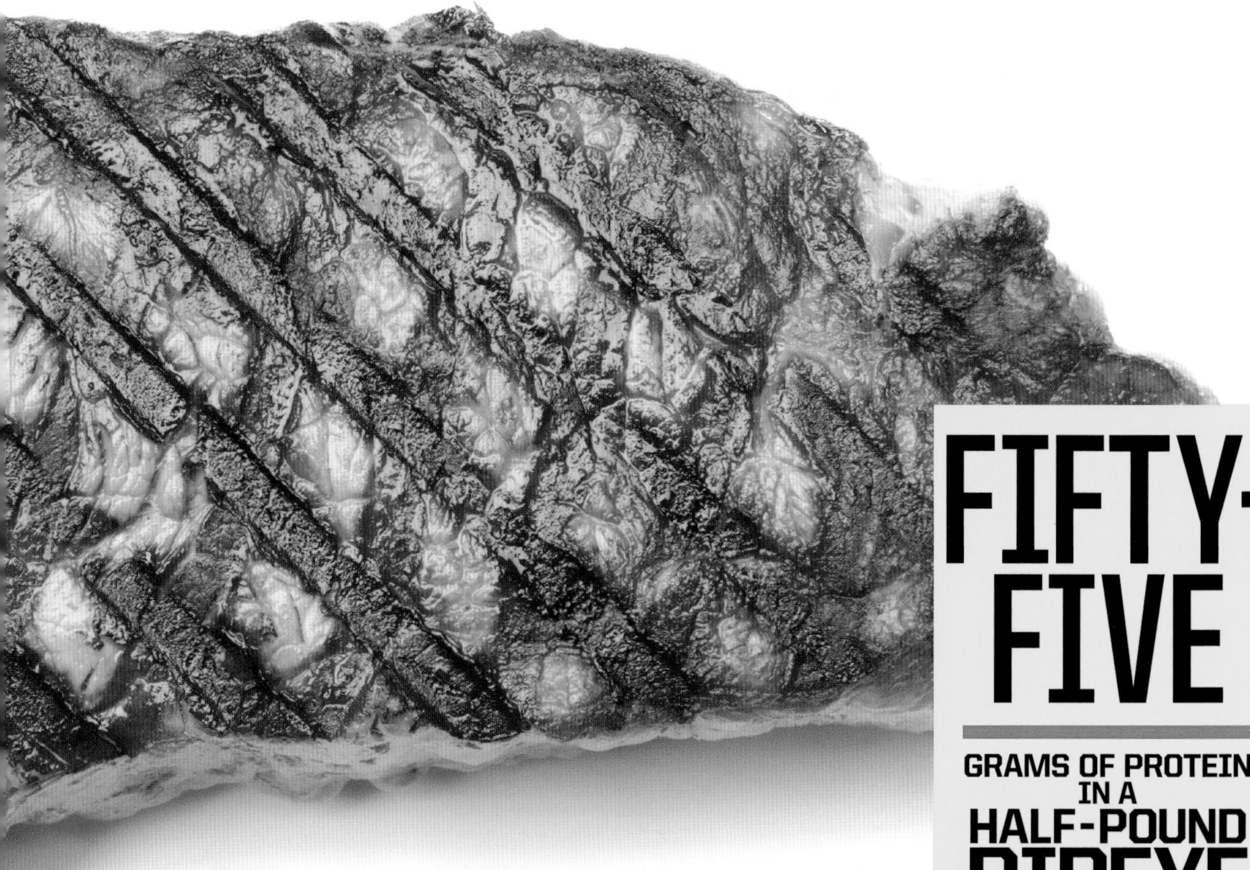

FIFTY-FIVE

GRAMS OF PROTEIN IN A HALF-POUND RIBEYE STEAK

DAY SNACK
cks light mozza-
string cheese
ge whole-wheat
bread
p hummus
pita into triangles
dip in hummus.)

NER
top sirloin steak
ge sweet potato
ps mixed green
l
sp olive oil and
gar-based dressing

HTTIME SNACK
ge apple
oop whey protein

TIME SNACK
ps popcorn
p low-fat cottage
se

Daily Totals: 3,333 calories, 300g protein, 335g carbs, 85g fat

For those training late at night...

BREAKFAST 1
½ cantaloupe
1 scoop whey protein
5g BCAAs

BREAKFAST 2
3 whole eggs
3 egg whites
2 cups cooked oatmeal
1 tbsp honey (add to oatmeal to sweeten)

LATE MORNING SNACK
1 cup reduced-fat Greek yogurt
½ scoop whey protein (your favorite flavor)
1 tsp honey
½ oz walnuts (7 halves), crushed
(Mix all ingredients in Greek yogurt and enjoy.)

LUNCH
5 oz can tuna (in water)
1 tbsp light mayonnaise
2 slices whole-wheat bread (or Ezekiel bread)

MIDDAY SNACK
3 sticks light mozzarella string cheese
1 large whole-wheat pita bread
¼ cup hummus
(Slice pita into triangles and dip in hummus.)

DINNER
8 oz top sirloin steak
1 large sweet potato
2 cups mixed green salad
2 tbsp olive oil and vinegar-based dressing

PRE-WORKOUT
1 large apple
1 scoop whey protein
5g BCAAs
1 dose creatine

WORKOUT

POST-WORKOUT
1 scoop whey protein
2 cups low-fat milk
10 Wonka Pixy Stix
5g BCAAs
1 dose creatine

BEDTIME SNACK
2 cups popcorn
1 cup low-fat cottage cheese

Daily Totals: 3,333 calories, 300g protein, 335g carbs, 85g fat

On rest days...

BREAKFAST 1
½ cantaloupe
1 scoop whey protein
5g BCAAs

BREAKFAST 2
3 whole eggs
3 egg whites
2 cups cooked oatmeal
1 tbsp honey (add to oatmeal to sweeten)

LATE-MORNING SNACK
1 cup reduced-fat Greek yogurt
½ scoop whey protein (your favorite flavor)
1 tsp honey
½ oz walnuts (7 halves), crushed
(Mix all ingredients in Greek yogurt and enjoy.)

LUNCH
5 oz can tuna (in water)
1 tbsp light mayonnaise
2 slices whole-wheat bread (or Ezekiel bread)

MIDDAY SNACK
3 sticks light mozzarella string cheese
1 large whole-wheat pita bread
¼ cup hummus
(Slice pita into triangles and dip in hummus.)

DINNER
8 oz top sirloin steak
1 large sweet potato
2 cups mixed green salad
2 tbsp olive oil and vinegar-based dressing

BEDTIME SNACK
2 cups popcorn
1 cup low-fat cottage cheese

Daily Totals: 2,750 calories, 245g protein, 255g carbs, 80g fat

Supplements

ONCE you've got solid training and nutrition programs in place, an equally solid supplement plan will only enhance your ability to get bigger, stronger, and leaner. As you've no doubt already seen, though, there's a lot of hype and misinformation swirling around the supplement industry. Before you fall for the hottest pre-workout supplement or some random ingredient that a fitness "guru" promises will make you grow muscle like body hair, take a long look at this guide, because all you need to get started on the right foot is here. And don't think we're about to sell you on a bunch of products you can't afford. Some of the most anabolic supplements can actually be obtained from whole foods. All of the supplements listed below, whether derived from whole foods or manufactured sources, help form the nutritional foundation upon which you'll build your best body ever.

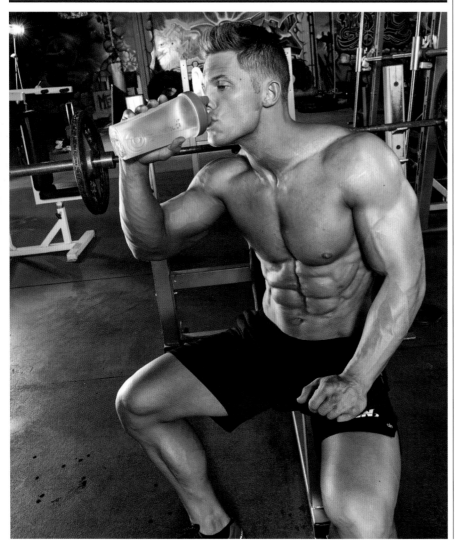

1 WHEY PROTEIN

Milk contains two primary types of protein: whey and casein. Whey is soluble an makes up 20% of milk protein, while cas makes up the remaining 80%. There's a r son whey is not only the best-selling prot powder on the market today, but the bes selling supplement, period: It builds lean muscle. No other protein digests as quic as whey, with its amino acids delivered to the bloodstream within 60–90 minutes.

This allows it to rapidly turn on muscle-protein synthesis for instigating muscle growth, which is especially important around workouts, when the muscles are primed for it. Another benefit of whey is it's the richest source of branched-chain amino acids (BCAAs) of all the nutritional proteins. The three aminos that make up BCAAs are the most critical for muscle growth and also provide the muscles with a fuel source (more on BCAAs shortly). Additionally, whey protein supplies speci peptides that relax the blood vessels to cause vasodilation, which gets more bloc flowing to the muscles and helps to deliv whey's amino acids to the muscles more quickly.

There's no more critical time to take wh than before and after workouts. In fact, research from Victoria University (Austra found that when subjects consumed whe protein, creatine, and glucose immediate before and after training for 10 weeks, they experienced an 80% greater increa in muscle mass and about a 30% greate increase in muscle strength than subject taking the same supplements in the morn and at night. They also lost body fat, whi the other group lost none. Furthermore, researchers from the University of Cope hagen found that subjects taking a prote and carbohydrate supplement immediately after workouts for 12 weeks gained significant muscle mass. The group takin the supplement immediately after worko also gained greater muscle strength.
DOSE: *Take around 20 grams of whey upon waking, within 30 minutes of your workouts, and then again within 30 minutes after your workouts.*

40 GRAMS

2 CREATINE

This is one of the most studied and effective supplements ever to hit the market. Research confirms that creatine can increase muscle mass by about 10 pounds and muscle strength by more than 10%. As you may have heard before, creatine does, in fact, increase the water weight inside muscles, pulling more fluid into the cells. But this fluid places a stretch on the membrane of muscle cells to signal an increase in muscle-protein synthesis, which results in real, long-term muscle growth. So don't listen to that know-it-all friend of yours who says that creatine just increases water weight. Creatine also provides the muscles a quick source of energy to fuel muscle contractions during workouts. In fact, creatine is a critical energy component of muscle cells. Having more of this energy available allows you to complete more reps with a given weight, which, over time, leads to gains in muscle strength and size.

DOSE: *Depending on the form of creatine you use, take 1–5 grams before and after workouts with whey protein. If you take creatine monohydrate, consider doing a loading phase for the first five to seven days. To do this, take 5 grams four to five times per day with meals. On workout days, make two of those doses pre- and post-workout. After the loading phase, stick with 5 grams, both pre- and post-workout.*

3 CASEIN PROTEIN

Unlike whey, casein is a very slow-digesting protein. It can take as long as seven hours to deliver all of its amino acids to your muscles. This is why we recommend that you get some form of casein before bedtime, whether that be from a protein shake or from whole foods like cottage cheese or Greek yogurt. Since casein is so slow to digest, many feel that it's a waste to take it around workouts. Yet numerous studies show that when you add casein to whey protein post-workout, muscle growth is increased beyond what's possible with whey alone—because while whey quickly starts muscle-protein synthesis, casein decreases muscle protein breakdown, which normally goes up after workouts. Since milk is a good source of casein, an easy way to add it post-workout is to mix whey in milk.

DOSE: *Add 20 grams of casein to your 20 of post-workout whey, and take 20 grams before bed. Other options include mixing whey in about two cups of low-fat milk or one cup of Greek yogurt, or drinking your whey shake with a cup of cottage cheese.*

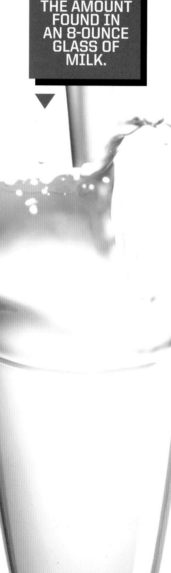

12 GRAMS OF SUGAR: THE AMOUNT FOUND IN AN 8-OUNCE GLASS OF MILK.

4 BCAAs

The branched-chain amino acids (BCAAs) include leucine, isoleucine, and valine. Of t three, leucine is the most critical for musc growth for two main reasons. First, it turn on muscle-protein synthesis in muscle cell which means increased potential for musc growth. The second reason is that leucine spikes levels of insulin, an anabolic hormo released from the pancreas that helps glu cose, amino acids, and creatine reach mus cells. Leucine also decreases muscle-prot breakdown and increases muscle-protein synthesis. That said, all three BCAAs are important because muscles can use them as direct energy sources, especially during workouts, which allows you to train harder with less fatigue. As a result, BCAAs are ic throughout the day for anyone looking to maximize gains. Take them before workou (for energy), after workouts (for better rec ery and muscle growth), and first thing in t morning (to stop muscle breakdown and p your body in an anabolic state).

DOSE: *Take 5 grams of BCAAs upon waking, within 30 minutes of starting your workouts, and then again within 30 minutes after your workouts.*

5 FAST CARBS

When you train, the main fuel source you burn is glucose, supplied by stored glycog within the muscle fibers. To have ample energy for your next workout, you need to restore that muscle glycogen as quickly a possible. Otherwise, the amount of glycog your muscles store for the next workout v be compromised, along with your energy a strength levels. After workouts, you need very fast-digesting (high-glycemic) carboh drate. The absolute fastest one is actually a complex carb called Vitargo, and the ne fastest is the sugar dextrose, which is act ally glucose—what your blood sugar and glycogen are composed of. If you don't wa to buy a dextrose/glucose powder supple ment to add to your post-workout shake, there are some candies that are mainly dextrose. Wonka Pixy Stix are pure dextrc and other good options include Wonka Bottle Caps, Wonka Sweetarts, and Harib gummy bears. Less sweet but almost as f is white bread and white potatoes.

DOSE: *Shoot for around 40–60 grams o fast-digesting carbs within 30 minutes after completing your workouts. If you us milk to mix your whey protein, remember that every cup of milk provides 12 grams of sugar. A good post-workout meal wou be one scoop of whey mixed in two cups milk plus 10–15 Wonka Pixy Stix.*

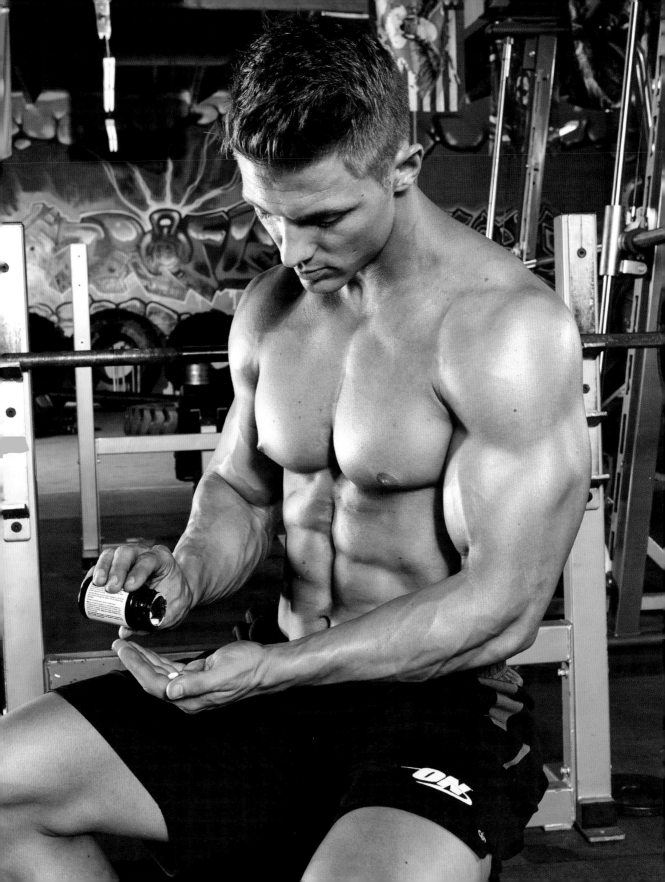

TIME OUT FOR MUSCLE

When it comes to designing training programs, we tend to focus on things like sets and reps, exercise order, and weights. The training variable that most often gets short shrift in this equation, however, is rest. Typically speaking, we don't give too much thought to the downtime during gym work. Taking a minute or two to muster the strength to knock out the next set is de rigueur for most gym rats; and while they may switch up the moves in their routines regularly, their rest periods remain static in perpetuity. It's time to rethink this strategy. Because, by playing with your rest times, you can improve the results of your training in terms of size, strength, and fat burning.

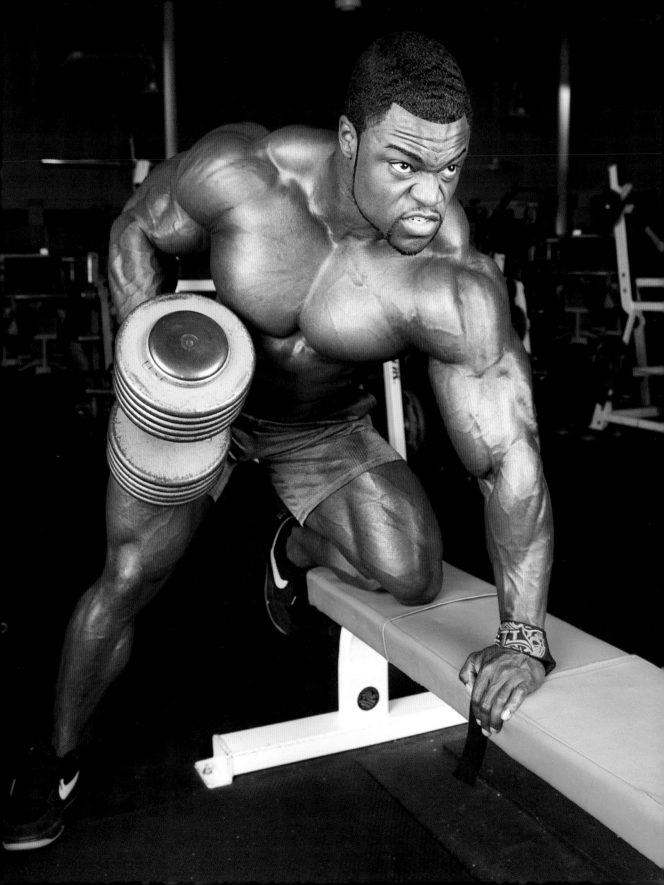

ON the one hand, longer rest periods equal more recovery time for fatigued muscles, which allows you to complete more reps on successive sets. The more reps you can do with a given weight, the stronger you'll become and the more muscle growth you'll stimulate. In fact, one study comparing a 2 ½-minute rest period versus a one-minute period between sets reported that novice lifters using the longer rest periods for 10 weeks increased their biceps size by 12%, while the shorter-resting group had only a 5% increase. However, novice lifters' muscles respond much differently to training than do those of the more experienced, so while this study may hold water for newbies, it's not as pertinent to seasoned gym rats.

When it comes to muscle hypertrophy and strength gains, other factors come into play, such as the biochemical changes in muscle that are triggered by fatigue. Such fatigue can lead to higher growth hormone and insulinlike growth factor-1 (IGF-1) levels, which can encourage better gains in muscle size. A recent study of trained male lifters in Brazil had one group training for eight weeks using an 8–10 rep range with a two-minute rest period between sets. Another group started out using a two-minute rest, then reduced it by 15 seconds each week until they were down to 30 seconds between sets in the eighth week. Researchers found that those dropping their rest times each week increased their arm size by 21% and leg size by 28%, while the group keeping rest constant at two minutes increased by only 14% and 19%, respectively. These results are mainly due to the fact that, as rest periods decrease, chemical stress increases. That chemical stress activates biochemical pathways that signal muscle growth, such as higher IGF-1 production, especially within muscle cells.

The gradual reduction in rest periods also trains the muscles to recover more quickly between sets, which results in greater strength and endurance. This ability to do more work in less time also triggers changes in the muscle that encourage growth. Fat burning is enhanced, too—yet another benefit of shortened rest periods.

These findings are precisely what the *M&F* Time Out program is based upon. You'll start off resting two minutes between sets, and each week you'll shave off 15 seconds until you're down to just 30 seconds of rest in Weeks 7 and 8. This will lead to more muscle, more endurance, more strength, and less fat—all while shortening your training time.

In addition to changing rest periods, this program delivers variety in every workout. Each exercise performed for a muscle group uses a different rep range; you'll start with

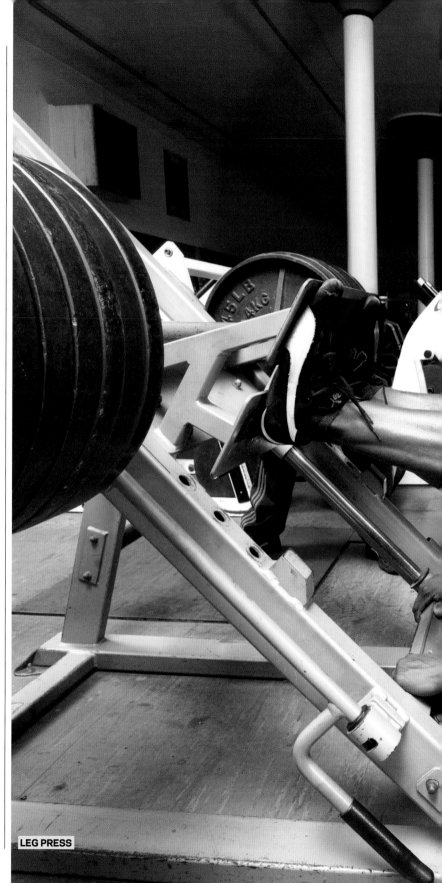

LEG PRESS

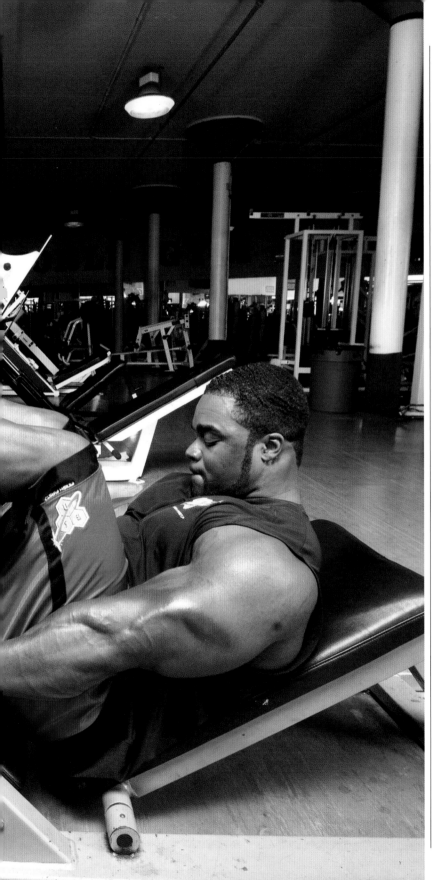

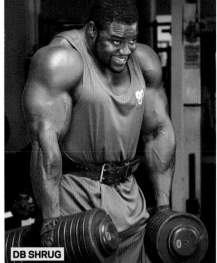

DB SHRUG

low reps and go up from there, which will bring you better gains in size, strength, and endurance, not to mention enhanced fat loss. Most muscle groups start off with a multijoint exercise or two, done with heavier weight and low reps (6–8 for the first exercise, 8–10 for the second) to place more overload on the target muscles before you get too fatigued. Then, you'll switch to single-joint moves, with higher reps using lighter weight (12–15 and 15–20 reps on the third and fourth exercises, respectively).

The program uses a four-day split in which opposing muscle groups are paired. For example, you'll train chest and biceps together in Workout 1 and back and triceps in Workout 4. This will ensure that smaller, assisting muscle groups don't get too fatigued early in the workout, before they're trained on their own. On Day 1, because biceps won't be affected much by your chest workout, they'll be relatively fresh when you train them; same goes for triceps on Day 4. With longer rest periods, this may not be as much of an issue. But once you get down to 30–45 seconds between sets, the intensity of your workouts will be such that you'll want to give every muscle group ample opportunity to recover and reap the strength, size, and fat-burning benefits of the Time Out program.

RUNNING OUT OF TIME

The rest periods between sets for each week of the Time Out program look like this:

WEEK	REST PERIOD BETWEEN SETS
1	2:00
2	1:45
3	1:30
4	1:15
5	1:00
6	0:45
7	0:30
8	0:30

DB LATERAL RAISE

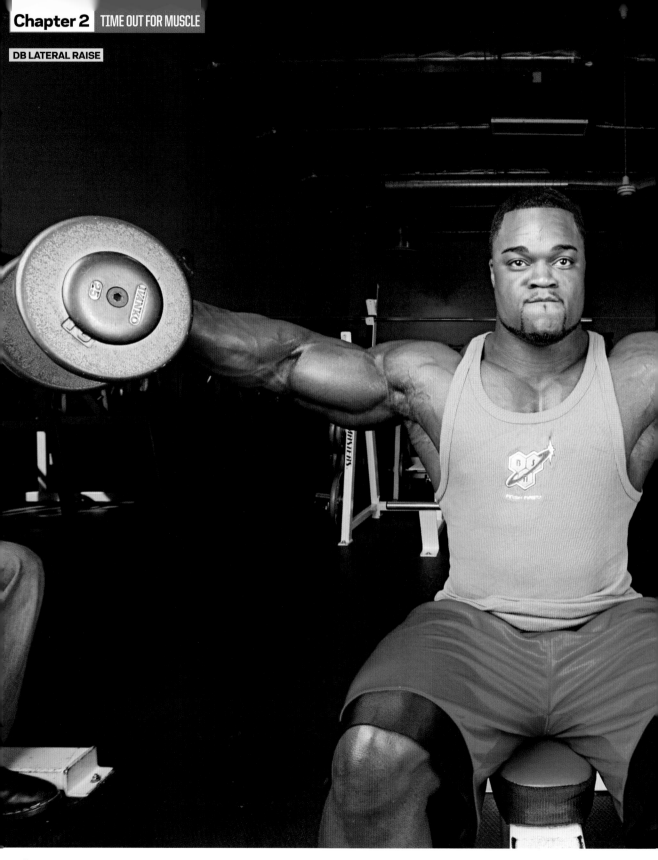

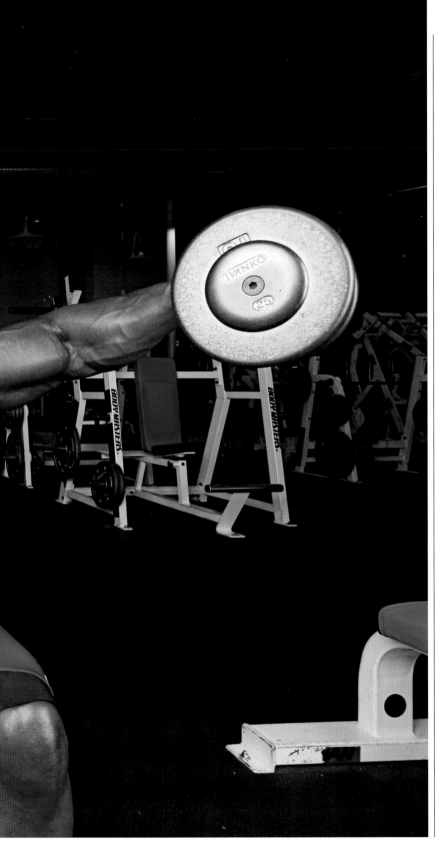

TIME OUT WORKOUTS
WEEKS 1, 3, 5, 7

WORKOUT 1: CHEST, BICEPS, ABS

EXERCISE	SETS	REPS
Bench Press	4	6-8
Incline Dumbbell Press	4	8-10
Incline Dumbbell Flye	3	12-15
Cable Crossover	3	15-20
Barbell Curl	3	6-8
Incline Dumbbell Curl	3	8-10
Lying Cable Concentration Curl	3	12-15
Dumbbell Hammer Curl	3	15-20
Rope Crunch	3	8-10
Hanging Leg Raise	3	12-15*
Oblique Crunch	3	15-20*

*Or as many as you can do

WORKOUT 2: LEGS, CALVES

EXERCISE	SETS	REPS
Squat	3	6-8
Leg Press	3	8-10
Lunge	3	12-15
Leg Extension	3	15-20
Romanian Deadlift	3	12-15
Leg Curl	3	15-20
Standing Calf Raise	4	12-15
Seated Calf Raise	4	15-20

WORKOUT 3: SHOULDERS, TRAPS, ABS

EXERCISE	SETS	REPS
Barbell Shoulder Press	4	6-8
Smith Machine Upright Row	4	8-10
Dumbbell Lateral Raise	3	12-15
Cable Rear-delt Flye	3	15-20
Barbell Shrug	3	6-8
Barbell Behind-the-back Shrug	3	8-10
Smith Machine Crunch	3	8-10
Plank	3	60-90 sec.
Reverse Crunch	3	15-20*

*Or as many as you can do

WORKOUT 4: BACK, TRICEPS, CALVES

EXERCISE	SETS	REPS
Dumbbell Bentover Row	4	6-8
Wide-grip Pulldown	4	8-10
Standing Pulldown	3	12-15
Dumbbell Straight-arm Pullback	3	15-20
Triceps Pressdown	3	12-15
Dumbbell Overhead Triceps Extension	3	15-20
Close-grip Bench Press	3	6-8
Dip	3	8-10
Seated Calf Raise	3	12-15
Leg-press Calf Raise	3	15-20

CABLE REAR-DELT FLYE

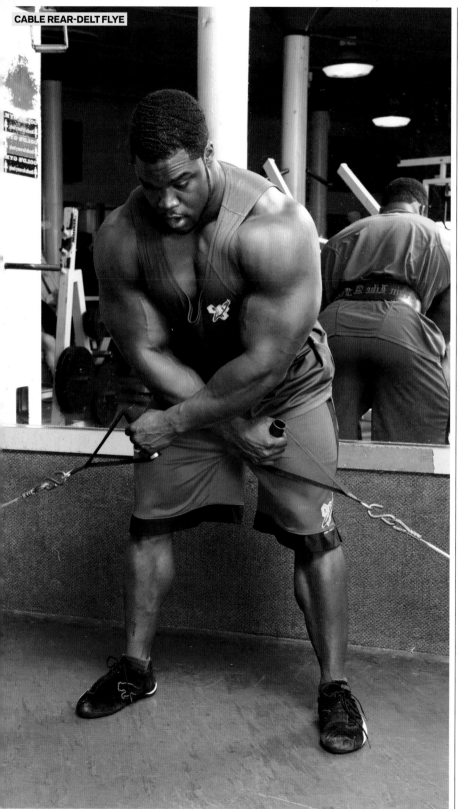

WEEKS 2, 4, 6, 8

WORKOUT 1: CHEST, BICEPS, ABS

EXERCISE	SETS	RE
Bench Press	4	6-
Incline Dumbbell Press	4	8-1
Low-pulley Cable Crossover	3	12-
Decline Flye	3	15-
Barbell Curl	3	6-
Incline Dumbbell Curl	3	8-1
Preacher Curl	3	12-
Rope-Cable Hammer Curl	3	15-
Rope Crunch	3	8-1
Hanging Leg Raise	3	12-
Oblique Crunch	3	15-

*Or as many as you can do

WORKOUT 2: LEGS, CALVES

EXERCISE	SETS	RE
Squat	3	6-
Leg Press	3	8-1
Lunge	3	12-
Leg Extension	3	15-
Romanian Deadlift	3	12-
Leg Curl	3	15-
Standing Calf Raise	4	12-
Seated Calf Raise	4	15-

WORKOUT 3: SHOULDERS, TRAPS, ABS

EXERCISE	SETS	RE
Barbell Shoulder Press	4	6-
Smith Machine Upright Row	4	8-1
Cable Lateral Raise	3	12-
Dumbbell Bentover Lateral Raise	3	15-
Barbell Shrug	3	6-
Dumbbell Shrug	3	8-1
Smith Machine Crunch	3	8-1
Plank	3	60- sec
Reverse Crunch	3	15-

*Or as many as you can do

WORKOUT 4: BACK, TRICEPS, CALVES

EXERCISE	SETS	RE
Dumbbell Bentover Row	4	6-
Wide-grip Pulldown	4	8-1
Inverted Row	3	12-
Straight-arm Pulldown	3	15-
Incline Dumbbell Kickback	3	12-
Cable Overhead Triceps Extension	3	15-
Close-grip Bench Press	3	6-8
Dip	3	8-1
Seated Calf Raise	3	12-
Leg-press Calf Raise	3	15-

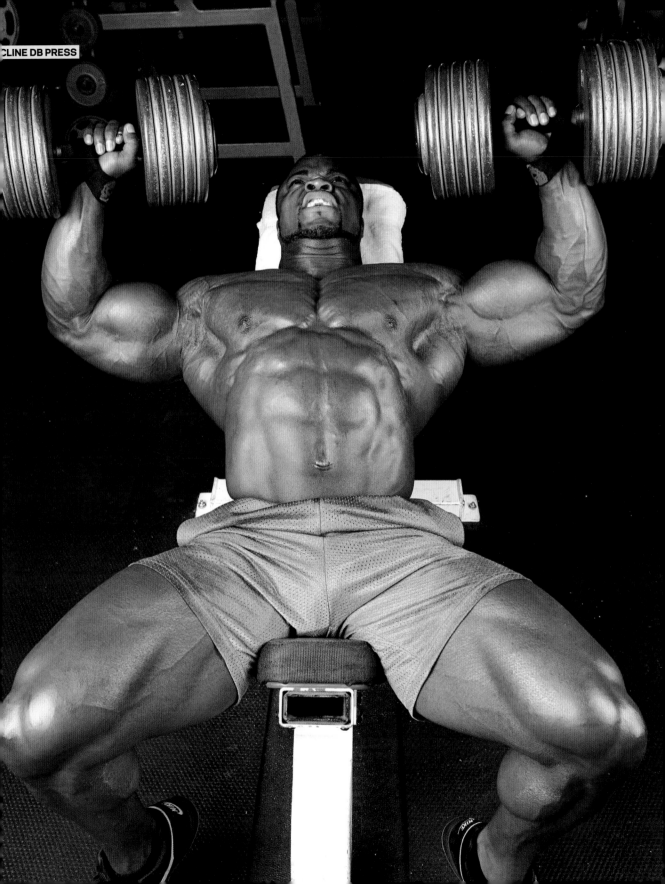

CLINE DB PRESS

If you don't like being in the gym, this program isn't for you. On the other hand, if you're a true M&Fer, you can't wait to get back in there after every session. Sometimes you even wish you could go back sooner. If this is your attitude, or you're a college student with an open class schedule or a guy who's currently between jobs and must vent his frustrations by lifting as much heavy iron as often as possible, two-a-days are exactly what you need.

DOUBLE

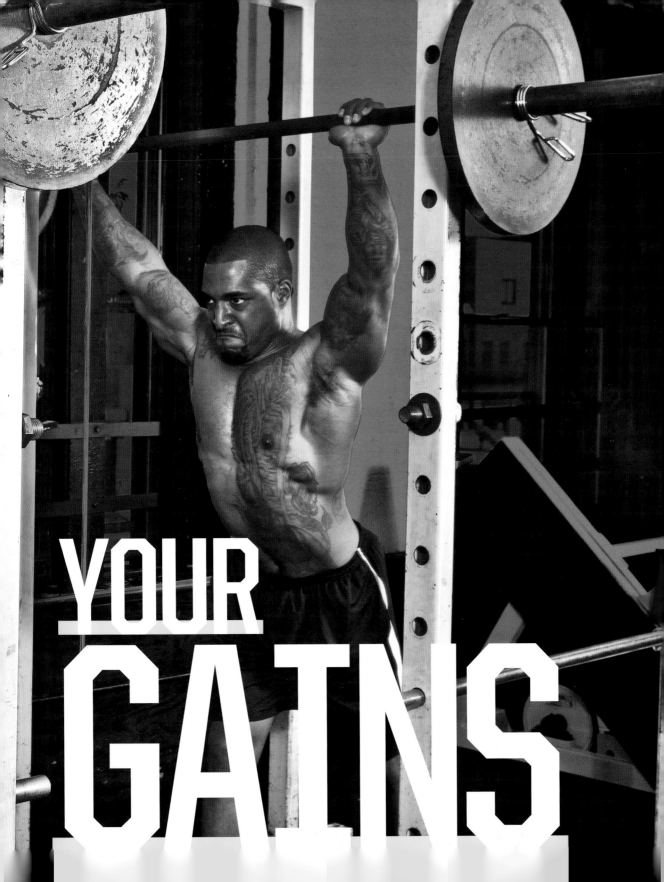

YOUR GAINS

THE FRUITS OF FREQUENCY

Training twice a day is a concept as old as bodybuilding itself but was popularized by Arnold more than anyone. He firmly believed his "double-split system" allowed him to separate himself from the pack and win his first Mr. Universe title. His rivals criticized it, saying it was too much training, and to their point, two-a-days have run many a lifter into the ground. But applied scientifically, there may be no better method for making big gains in a short period.

The reason is frequency. Provided you can recover from each session, the more often you train a body part, the faster you can deliver a growth stimulus and the sooner your muscles will respond. Training your chest so hard that it takes a whole week to recover before you can hit it again isn't as effective as hitting it light one day and then hard three days later. That's two chest-building workouts in one week, so you essentially double the stimulus.

Keep your sessions six to eight hours apart, and get as much sleep as possible at night. Good nutrition is part of recovery, so eat at least one gram of protein per pound of your body weight daily.

You'll train one or two body parts per session. The morning session will be light and the evening one heavy (or vice versa). The sessions won't be very long—you should be out of the gym in 45 minutes. The exception to this is Day 1's workout. Your leg blitz is so intense that you won't be doing a second session that day. You won't miss it.

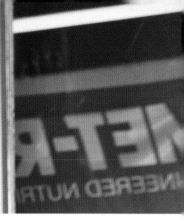

DOUBLE YOUR GAINS WORKOUTS

DIRECTIONS:

SPLIT: Each workout day comprises an a.m. and p.m. session except Day 1. We suggest you set up your training week as follows: Monday, Day 1; Tuesday, off; Wednesday, Day 2; Thursday, Day 3; Friday, off; Saturday, Day 4; Sunday, Day 5. Take that following Monday off and begin the cycle again Tuesday. Do no cardio.
HOW TO DO IT: Perform the exercises as straight sets. Note that some of the exercises need to be done in a specific way.

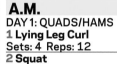

A.M.

DAY 1: QUADS/HAMS

1 Lying Leg Curl
Sets: 4 Reps: 12

2 Squat
Sets: 4 Reps: 12, 10, 8, 6
Increase the weight each set but stay two reps short of failure on all sets.

3 Leg Press w/ Bands
Sets: 4 Reps: 8
Use two pro mini-bands if you're new to banded exercises, or two monster mini-bands if you're more experienced. Fold each band over itself so you have two loops, and hook one end on the plate-loading peg of the leg press station on each side. Hook the other end on the bottom handle. Perform leg presses as normal.

4 Hack Squat
Sets: 3 Reps: 15
Use a hack squat machine and stand with your feet shoulder-width apart on the foot plate. Squat down as deeply as you can.

A.M.

DAY 2: CHEST (LIGHT)

1 Neutral-grip Machine Press
Sets: 6 Reps: 8
Use a chest press machine and grab the handles with your palms facing each other. Feel the stretch at the bottom of the movement and flex your pecs hard after lockout.

2 Pec Minor Dip
Sets: 3 Reps: 5
Suspend yourself over the parallel bars of a dip station. Keeping your elbows straight, pull your shoulder blades together so your torso moves closer to the floor. Spread your shoulders to come back up.

3 Ladder Pushup
Sets: 1 Reps: To failure
Place a bar on the bottom rung of a power

rack and perform as many pushups as possible. Immediately move it up about a foot to a higher rung and rep out again. Raise the bar one more time another 12–18 inches and rep out again. If your gym has one, use a cambered bar (it's curved in the middle, so you can lower your chest farther down).

P.M.
DAY 2: SHOULDERS (HEAVY)
1 Heavy Lateral Swing
Sets: 4 Reps: 35
Hold a heavy dumbbell in each hand (more than you'd use for a strict lateral raise) and use momentum to swing the weights away from your sides. The range of motion is small. Keep a slight bend in your elbows and tilt your head back (to minimize trap involvement).
2 Cage Press
Sets: 4 Reps: 6
Stand in a power rack and hold the bar at shoulder level with hands shoulder-width apart. Split your stance so one leg is in front of the other. Press the bar into the supports of the rack and upward so it scrapes along the metal. Keep the bar in contact with the frame as you lower it.

A.M.
DAY 3: UPPER BACK
1 Meadows Row
Sets: 3 Reps: 8
Wedge a barbell in the corner of a room and load one sleeve with small plates. Stand with one leg in front of the other and bend over at the hips to grab the end of the bar with an overhand grip. Row the bar to your side.
2 Dumbbell Pullover
Sets: 3 Reps: 12
Lie back on a bench holding a dumbbell with both hands. Press up, locking your arms, until the weight is above your face, then lower it behind your head with arms nearly straight until you feel a stretch in your lats.
3 Medium-grip Pullup
Sets: 3 Reps: 12
4 Stretcher
Sets: 3 Reps: 10
Attach a V-grip handle to the pulley of a lat-pulldown station. Place one foot on the seat with your leg straight. Allow the weight to pull your arms straight over your head and stretch your lats. Now lean back and pull the handle to your sternum.
5 Barbell Shrug
Sets: 2 Reps: 15
Hold the top position for three seconds on each rep.

P.M.
DAY 3: HAMS/LOWER BACK
1 Seated Leg Curl
Sets: 3 Reps: 15
Perform these as a warmup. Do not go heavy or to failure.
2 Stiff-leg Deadlift
Sets: 4 Reps: 15, 12, 9, 6

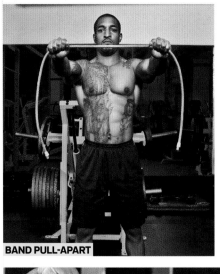

BAND PULL-APART

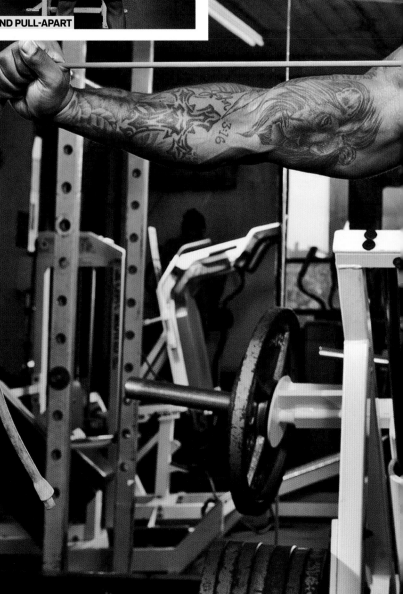

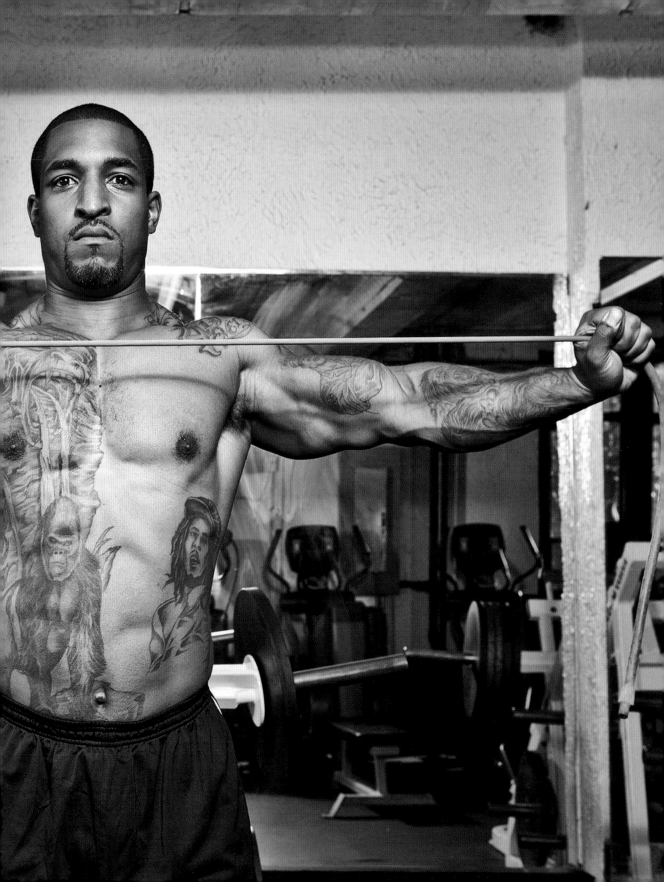

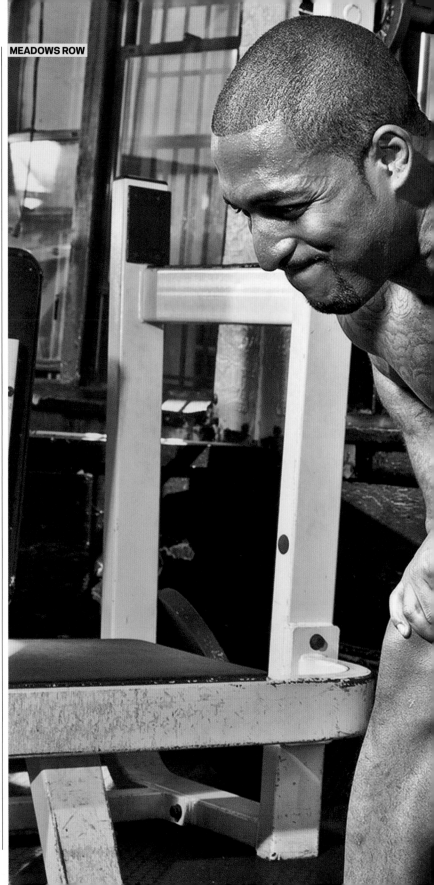
MEADOWS ROW

Keep a slight bend in your knees. Come up only three quarters of the way from the bottom on each rep.

3 Deficit Deadlift
Sets: 5 Reps: 5

Stack some plates on the floor or stand on a block or step so that you're about six inches above the floor. Perform the deadlift from this elevation. Choose a weight that lets you perform every rep explosively.

4 Reverse Hyperextension
Sets: 3 Reps: 12

Set an adjustable bench to an incline and lie down on it facing the seat (so your legs hang off the head of the bench). Squeeze your glutes and raise your legs up until they're in line with your body.

A.M.

DAY 4: CHEST (HEAVY)

1 Decline Dumbbell Press
Sets: 3 Reps: 8

The decline should be slight. Flex your chest at the top of each rep for two seconds.

2 Incline Bench Press
Sets: 4 Reps: 12, 10, 8, 6

Stop each rep one to two inches short of your chest and do not lock out any reps. Keep tension on your chest.

3 Reverse Band Bench Press
Sets: 6 Reps: 5

Use two light jump stretch bands. Attach one to the top beam on each side of a power rack, or to the safety rods set at the highest level in the rack. Loop the other end of the bands onto the sleeves of the bar. Perform the bench press, allowing the bands to unload the weight at the bottom of the movement.

P.M.

DAY 4: SHOULDERS (LIGHT)

1 Machine Rear-delt Flye
Sets: 4 Reps: 25

Hold the contracted position for one second.

2 Band Pull-apart
Sets: 3 Reps: 15

Hold a band at arm's length in front of you. Keeping your elbows straight, pull your arms backward as in a rear-delt flye. You'll stretch the band two or three times its resting length. Hold the contracted position for a second.

3 Six-way Shoulder Raise
Sets: 4 Reps: 10

Sit on a bench holding a light dumbbell in each hand and perform a lateral raise. Move your arms in front of your body so you're in the top position of a front raise. Now raise the weights straight overhead. Lower the weights back to the front raise, move them out to your sides (the top of the lateral raise again), and then lower. That's one rep.

A.M.

DAY 5: BICEPS/ CALVES

1 Seated Dumbbell Curl
Sets: 3 Reps: 12

Keep your palms turned up on every rep and

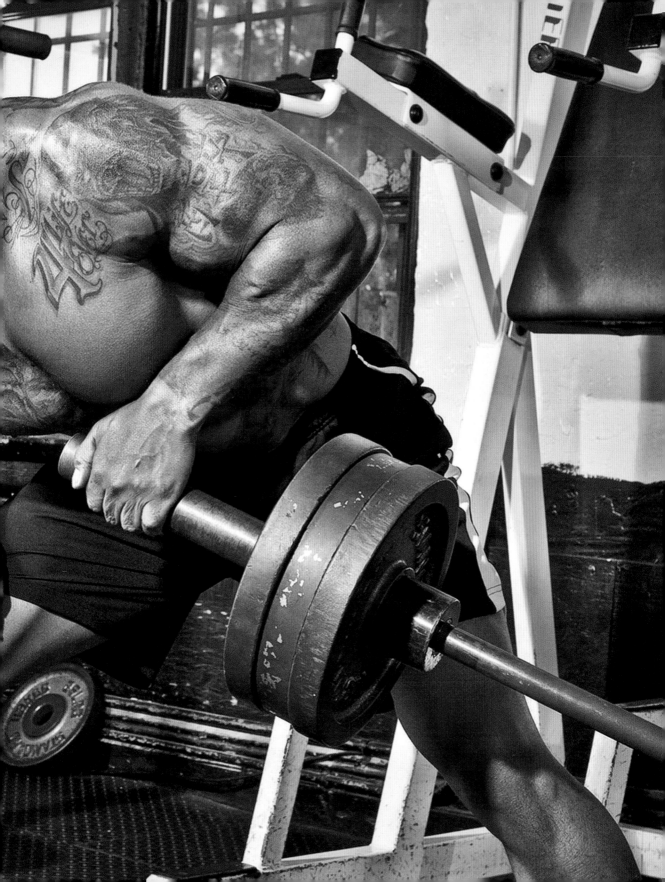

take three seconds to lower each rep.

2 EZ-bar Preacher Curl
Sets: 3 Reps: 8
Flex the biceps at the top of each rep.

3 Cross-body Hammer Curl
Sets: 3 Reps: 10 (each arm)
Hold a dumbbell in each hand and perform a hammer curl across your body. Your right hand will come up to your left shoulder and vice versa. Squeeze the dumbbell handles hard throughout.

4 Incline Concentration Curl
Sets: 3 Reps: 10
Set an adjustable bench to an incline and lie facedown on it with a dumbbell in each hand. Keeping your palms turned toward the ceiling, curl the weights up to your shoulders without moving your upper arms forward. Press the dumbbells together as you curl.

5 Calf Raise on Leg Press w/ Bands
Sets: 3 Reps: As many as possible
Place your toes on the foot plate of a leg press machine and let the weight extend your ankles. Press your toes hard into the plate, flexing your ankles to push the weight up.

6 Seated Calf Raise
Sets: 2 Reps: 12
Feel the stretch at the bottom and hold the top position for two seconds.

P.M.
DAY 5: TRICEPS/ABS
1 Rope Pushdown
Sets: 4 Reps: 12
2 Dip Between Benches
Sets: 3 Reps: To failure
Place your hands on a bench behind you; your feet on another bench in front of you.
3 EZ-bar Incline Extension
Sets: 3 Reps: 15
Set an adjustable bench to an incline and lie back against it. Grab an EZ-bar with an overhand, shoulder-width grip and raise it over your head. Keeping your upper arms in place, bend your elbows and lower the bar until it's behind your head. Extend your elbows to raise it back up.
4 V-Up
Sets: 4 Reps: To failure
Lie on your back on the floor with your legs straight and arms pointed to the wall behind your head. Then simultaneously raise your legs overhead while reaching for your feet with your arms. Your body should form a V shape at the top.
5 Banded Ab Crunch
Sets: 4 Reps: 10
Loop a band around the top of a power rack and grab an end in each hand. Hold the band by your ears and stand with your feet wider than shoulder width. Push your hips back and crunch your torso down. Push your hips forward when you come up.

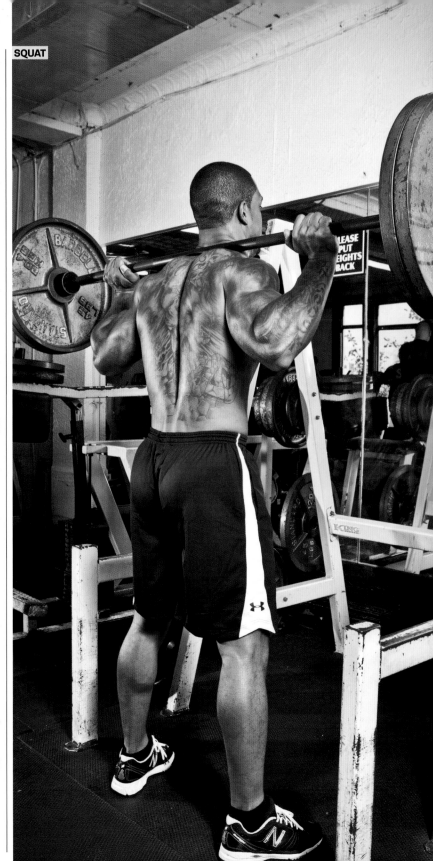

SQUAT

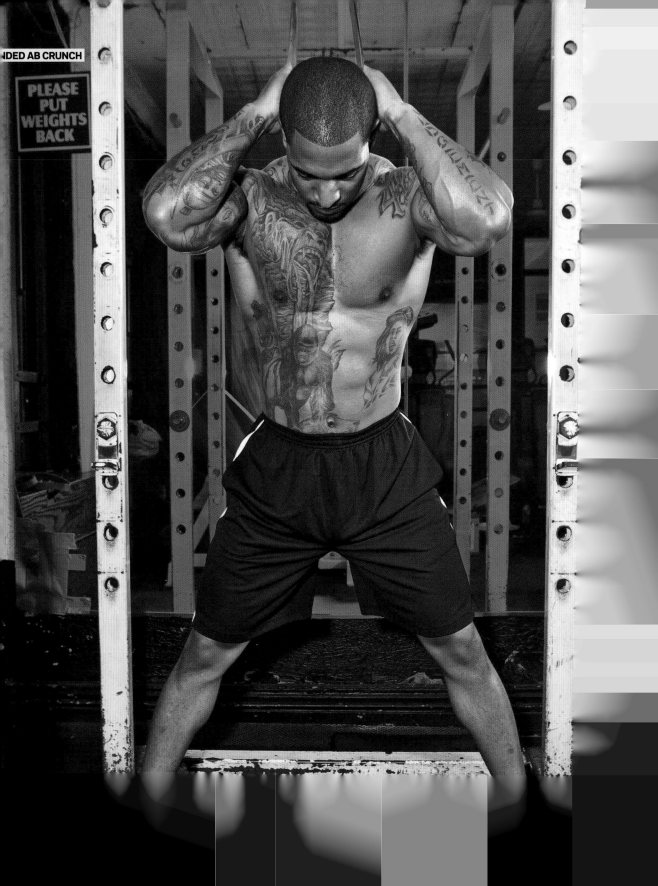

PLEASE
PUT
WEIGHTS
BACK

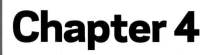

Chapter 4

YOUR BODY IS YOUR GREATEST PROJECT. WE'VE GOT THE BLUEPRINT TO GET YOU BIGGER AND STRONGER THAN EVER BEFORE.
BY CJ MURPHY, FOUNDER OF TOTAL PERFORMANCE SPORTS AND A FORMER NATIONAL CHAMPION POWERLIFTE

OVERHEAD SQUAT
Key Points:

Keep the shoulders back so that the bar is behind your head, not over it, and keep your chin tucked in slightly.

Sit back into the squat as you normally would, keeping the movement slow and controlled, and pause at the bottom to find your balance.

Get your hips below your knees.

BUILD BRUTE STRENGTH

Look around. There are countless articles in magazines and online about gaining size and strength. Everyone wants to get strong, and everyone wants to add muscle, but most don't achieve the goal. Why? A number of reasons, including ridiculous exercise selection, poor programming, and—from what I've seen as a coach for almost 25 years—bad form.

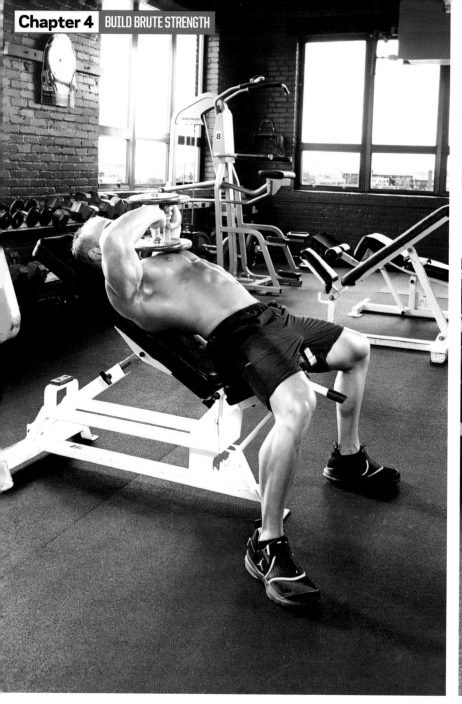

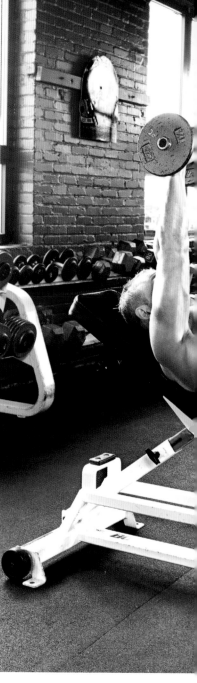

If you're willing to do the hard work and make the commitment to using perfect form, I've got the ultimate plan for you: an eight-week guide to getting stronger than you ever thought you could.

It's a simple plan based on compound movements, high-repetition heavy lifting, and maximum-effort training. Throw in the right assistance work and you've got a plan for success.

Our goals for the next eight weeks are massive increases in strength throughout the whole body, and enhanced muscle size. Don't worry if you don't get superjacked right away. You'll add some muscle now, but the real size will come later on, as you begin to use the newfound strength developed with this program.

Strength is the basis for everything we do in the gym and in life. If you want to get huge, you've got to get strong. Raising your limit strength (the amount you can lift once) allows you to handle a heavier submaximal weight for more reps. Let me illustrate:

Generally, low reps build strength and high reps build size, right? Sort of. Well, in this program, you'll be doing a blend of both, but you'll also be doing heavy weights for higher reps.

Using heavy weights for high reps on basic exercises causes a large release of growth hormone in your body and also increases testosterone levels. It's the cheapest growth hormone and testosterone-boosting supplement available.

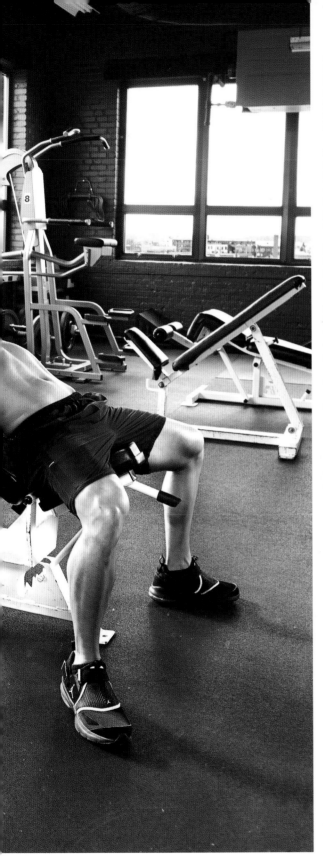

STRENGTH BY DESIGN

Let's talk about the program. You'll be working brutally hard in three-week blocks, then de-loading on the fourth week, a period of lighter training with less volume. It all begins again in Week 5 with a new plan of attack for three weeks before dropping back for another de-loading phase.

Don't underestimate the importance of de-loading—if you follow the program with the correct intensity, you'll need it. You won't get weak though; you'll actually get stronger because of it. Your body has different types of muscle fibers, with subdivisions of those different types. The very explosive ones fatigue quickly and take a long time to recover. By de-loading on your fourth week, you give your central nervous system (CNS) and the explosive fibers a chance to rest and regenerate.

In the same spirit, this program calls for only three days of training per week. You'll be doing a lot of volume and tonnage in your workouts, so you need to allow for that when programming, and make sure you get adequate rest to prevent overtraining. Don't add days—add intensity to each session.

I've given you a lower-body strength day (Day 1), an upper-body strength day with a few assistance exercises (Day 2), and a full-body assistance day at the end of the week (Day 3). This allows you to train hard, recover, then do it again, creating strength gains but also making sure you have enough energy to bring up weak points on assistance day.

You'll also be doing supersets, because I believe in training economy and density. Density means cramming as much work into a given time period as possible. The idea is to get into the gym, get your results, and get out.

In the plan as a whole, you'll notice that as the weeks go on, both total work (volume) and amount of weight lifted decrease. For instance, in Week 1 on squats, if you use 225 pounds for all sets, it works out to 13,500 total pounds lifted; in Week 3, if you use 275 pounds for all sets, you'll have lifted 6,875 pounds. This might seem backward to you, but as the weight increases, the load on your CNS increases as well. You can't expect progress if you're burning out your CNS. Dropping the volume as nervous system demand increases allows you to fire more motor units to move more weight.

As you progress from week to week, some weeks you'll see an increase in assistance work as total volume goes down on main lifts. This goes back once again to nervous system demands. Your assistance work doesn't require nearly as much neurological activity, and therefore is less demanding of your body's recovery systems. You can handle more assistance work, and you'll benefit greatly from it. Again, don't add in more exercises or sets. Just stick to the plan.

TATE PRESS
Key Points:
Lie on an incline bench holding two dumbbells just as you would for a dumbbell bench press.

Flare your elbows directly out to the sides to lower the weights to your chest with your palms facing your feet.

When the plates of the dumbbells touch your chest, reverse the motion to press the weights back up.

45-DEGREE BARBELL ROW

Key Points:
Keep the torso locked in place at a 45-degree angle with the floor.
Keep your weight over your heels, and keep your lats and shoulder blades pulled down.
Drag the bar up your thighs to your lower abs.

MURPH'S STRENGTH PROGRAM

1
Precede all workouts with a 5- to 10-minute warmup of your choice. A dynamic warmup and soft tissue work (like foam rolling) is preferred.

2
When only a number is given for reps (i.e., 50 reps or 100 reps), do as many sets as it takes to achieve the rep count, resting as little as possible. Do a set to near (not complete) failure, rest, and keep going.

3
On warmups for main lifts (squats, deadlifts, presses), stick with 1–3 reps. For example, if your first work set in the squat uses 315 pounds, warmups will look like this: Bar x 5, 95 x 3, 135 x 3, 185 x 3, 225 x 2, 275 x 1.

4
Visit CJ Murphy's YouTul channel (*youtube.com /total performance1*) t see videos of selected exercises in this progran Click on "Playlists" the select "Exercise of the Month Archives."

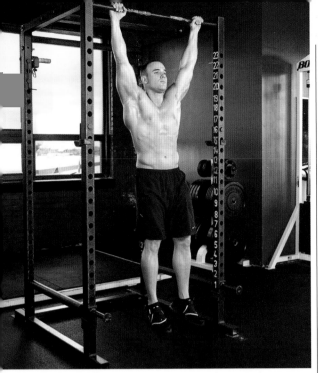
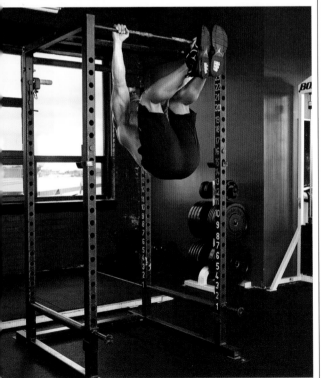

WEEKS 1-3

DAY 1

EXERCISE	WEEK 1 SETS/REPS	WEEK 2 SETS/REPS	WEEK 3 SETS/REPS
Squat	5/12	5/8	5/5
Deadlift	5/5	5/3	3/3
Back Extension	50 reps	75 reps	100 reps
Ab Wheel	50 reps	75 reps	100 reps

DAY 2

EXERCISE	WEEK 1 SETS/REPS	WEEK 2 SETS/REPS	WEEK 3 SETS/REPS
Incline Bench Press	5/12	5/8	5/5
Overhead Press	5/12	5/8*	4/6*
45-Degree Barbell Row	4/10-12**	3/8-10***	4/6-8***
Dumbbell Side Bend	5/5	4/6	5/3

*Do 5 pullups between each set. If you can't do a pullup, use an elastic band for assistance.

**Do 6-8 towel pullups between each set in Weeks 2 and 3, respectively, looping a towel over the pullup bar and holding onto it instead of the bar. If you can't do a towel pullup, use an elastic band for assistance.

***In between sets do 8-10 reps of barbell shrugs (no wrist straps) in Week 2. Do 6-8 reps in Week 3.

DAY 3 (FULL-BODY ASSISTANCE)

EXERCISE	WEEK 1 SETS/REPS	WEEK 2 SETS/REPS	WEEK 3 SETS/REPS
Walking Lunge	5/12* per leg	5/10 per leg	4/8* per leg
Dip	50 reps**	75 reps**	100 reps**
Keystone Deadlift	4/10-12***	3/8-10***	2/8-10***
One-Arm Dumbbell Row	4/10-12	3/8-10	2/12-15
Tate Press	3/10-12****	3/8-10****	2/12-15****
Turkish Get-up	3/3 per side	3/5 per side	5/3 per side

*Do 5, 6, or 8 pullups between each set in Weeks 1, 2, and 3, respectively.

**Do 5, 6, or 8 weighted situps between each set in Weeks 1, 2, and 3, respectively.

***Do 5, 6, or 10 inverted rows between each set in Weeks 1, 2, and 3, respectively.

****Do 10-12, 8-10, or 12-15 hammer curls between each set in Weeks 1, 2, and 3, respectively.

WEEK 4 (DE-LOAD)

DAY 1

EXERCISE	SETS/REPS
Squat	5/5*
One-leg Romanian Deadlift	3/6 per leg
One-leg Back Extension	2/10-12 per leg
Hanging Leg Raise	3/AMAP**

*Use 55% of your heaviest weight from Week 3.

**AMAP: As many [reps] as possible.

DAY 2

EXERCISE	SETS/REPS
Incline Bench Press	5/5*
Dumbbell Overhead Press	3/10-12**
T-bar Row	3/10-12
One-Arm Deadlift	3/5 per arm

*Use 55% of your heaviest weight from Week 3.

**Do 5 pullups between each set with a one-second hold at the top and middle of each rep.

NGING LEG RAISE

Points:

rt the movement with a straight-leg ab crunch, shortening the distance ween your ribs and your hips.

er engaging your abs with the crunch, bring your legs up as high as you , rounding your back in the process.

ging leg raises can be done either with ab straps or hanging from a up bar (the latter also improves grip strength).

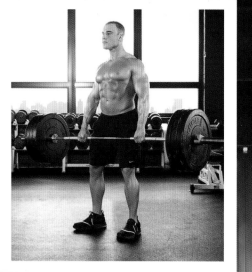

KEYSTONE DEADLIFT
Key Points:
Keep the chest up and butt pushed out and the back arched throughout the movement. Don't lose this position.
Initiate the movement by pushing the hips back and dragging the weight down your thighs until your knuckles touch your kneecaps.
To come up, squeeze your glutes.

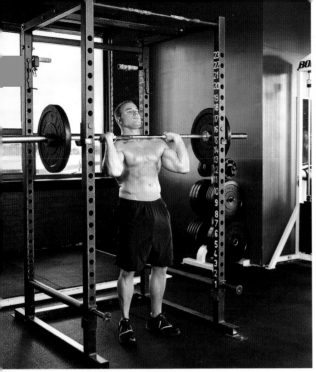

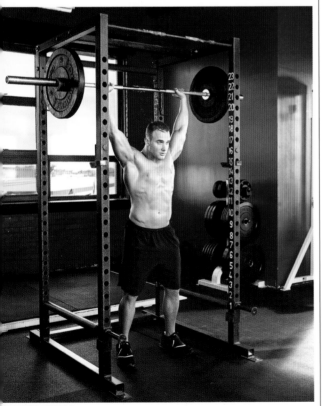

DAY 3 (FULL-BODY ASSISTANCE)

EXERCISE	SETS/REPS
Overhead Squat	3/6*
Dip	50 reps**
Turkish Get-up	5/5

*Do 5 pullups between each set of overhead squats.
**Do 8 situps between each set of dips.

WEEKS 5-7

DAY 1

EXERCISE	WEEK 5 SETS/REPS	WEEK 6 SETS/REPS	WEEK 7 SETS/REPS
Squat	5/5*	5/3	Max single***
Deadlift	5/5**	5/3	2-rep Max***
Weighted Back Extension	50 reps	60 reps	50 reps
Ab Wheel****	75 reps	100 reps	85 reps

*Go 5-10% heavier than in Week 3.
**Go 5% heavier than in Week 3.
***Work up gradually to your max weight on the squat and deadlift, respectively, using the warmup progression described above. When you get to your max weight, do 1 final set of 1 rep for squats and 1 final set of 2 reps for deadlifts.
****Pause for one second at the fully extended position on all reps.

DAY 2

EXERCISE	WEEK 5 SETS/REPS	WEEK 6 SETS/REPS	WEEK 7 SETS/REPS
Overhead Press	5/5*	5/3	Max
Close-grip Incline Press	4/12**	4/8-10**	4/6-8**
45-Degree Barbell Row	3/12-15***	4/10-12***	3/6-8***
Farmer's Walk****	6/100 feet	6/100 feet	4/100 feet

*Go 5-10% heavier than in Week 3.
**Do 10 towel pullups between each set in Week 5 and 12 in Weeks 6-7.
***Do 12-15, 10-12, or 6-8 reps of barbell shrugs (no wrist straps) between each set in weeks 5, 6, and 7, respectively.
****Increase weight for Week 6; in Week 7, stick with the same weight or go lighter.

DAY 3 (FULL-BODY ASSISTANCE)

EXERCISE	WEEK 5 SETS/REPS	WEEK 6 SETS/REPS	WEEK 7 SETS/REPS
Good Morning	5/12-15*	4/8-10*	3/8-10*
Weighted Dip	50** reps	60** reps	70** reps
Step-up	4/8-12***	3/12-15***	3/8-10***
One-arm Dumbbell Row	4/12-15	4/8-12	4/6-8
Tate Press****	4/12-15	4/8-12	3/6-8
Turkish Get-up	5/5 per side	5/3 per side	3/3 per side

*Do 10 or 12 pullups between each set in Weeks 5 and 6, respectively, and as many pullups as possible between each set in Week 7.
**Do 10 or 12 weighted situps between each set in Weeks 5 and 6, respectively; in Week 7, use a heavy weight and do 6 reps between each set.
***Do 10 or 12 inverted rows between each set in Weeks 5 and 6, respectively, and as many as possible between each set in Week 7; do the prescribed number of step-ups per leg.
****Do 12-15, 8-12, or 6-8 hammer curls between each set in Weeks 5, 6, and 7, respectively.

ERHEAD PRESS
Points:
ss the bar slightly back behind your head at the top.
en the bar passes your face, drive your head forward and through.
celerate the bar faster as it gets higher, and drive your knuckles
ard the ceiling.

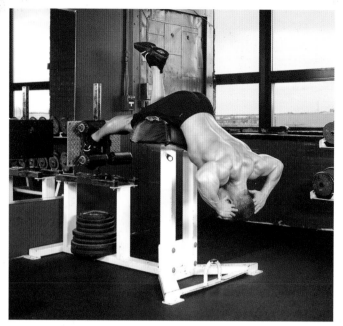

WEEK 8 (DE-LOAD)

DAY 1

EXERCISE	SETS/REPS
Squat	5/5*
Deadlift	3/5**
One-leg Back Extension	3/12 per l
Lying Leg Raise	50 reps

*Use 55% of your 1-rep max.
**Use 45% of your 2-rep max.

DAY 2

EXERCISE	SETS/REP
Overhead Press	5/5*
Incline Dumbbell Press	3/12
Pullup	3/AMAP*
Farmer's Walk	4/100 feet

*Use 55% of your 1-rep max on the overhead press.
**AMAP: As many [reps] as possible.

DAY 3 (FULL-BODY ASSISTANCE)

EXERCISE	SETS/REP
Overhead Squat	3/6-8
Dip	50 reps
Step-up	3/8-10 per
One-arm Dumbbell Row	3/12-15
Turkish Get-up	3/5 per si

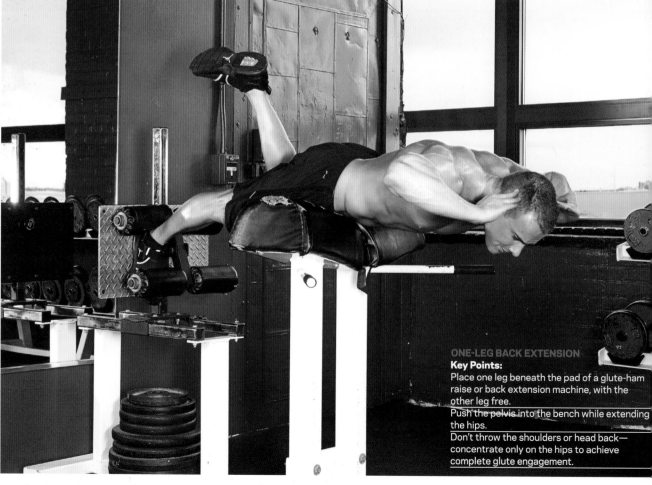

ONE-LEG BACK EXTENSION
Key Points:
Place one leg beneath the pad of a glute-ham raise or back extension machine, with the other leg free.
Push the pelvis into the bench while extending the hips.
Don't throw the shoulders or head back—concentrate only on the hips to achieve complete glute engagement.

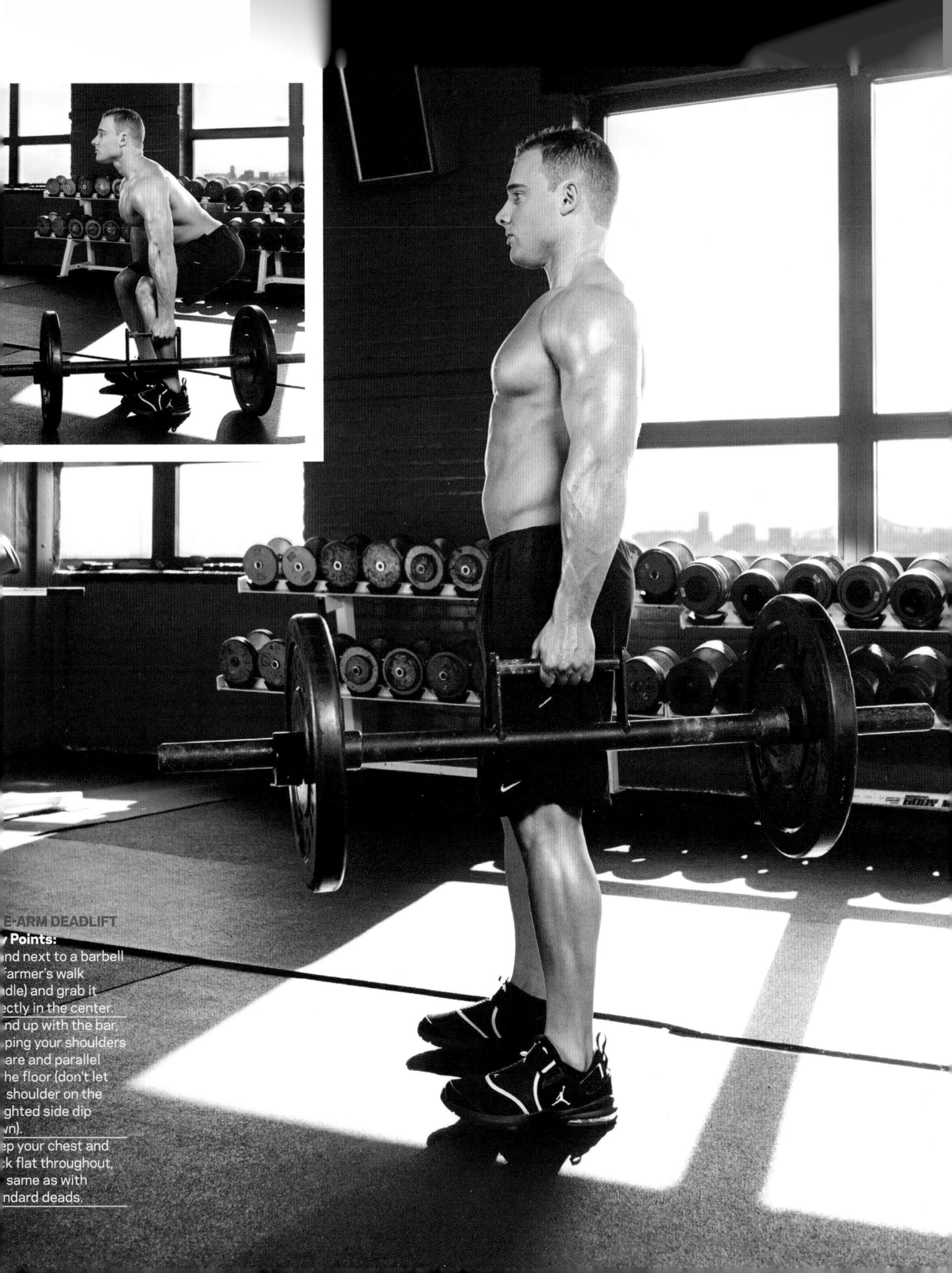

E-ARM DEADLIFT

Points:

nd next to a barbell
armer's walk
dle) and grab it
ectly in the center.
nd up with the bar,
ping your shoulders
are and parallel
he floor (don't let
shoulder on the
ghted side dip
n).

ep your chest and
k flat throughout,
same as with
ndard deads.

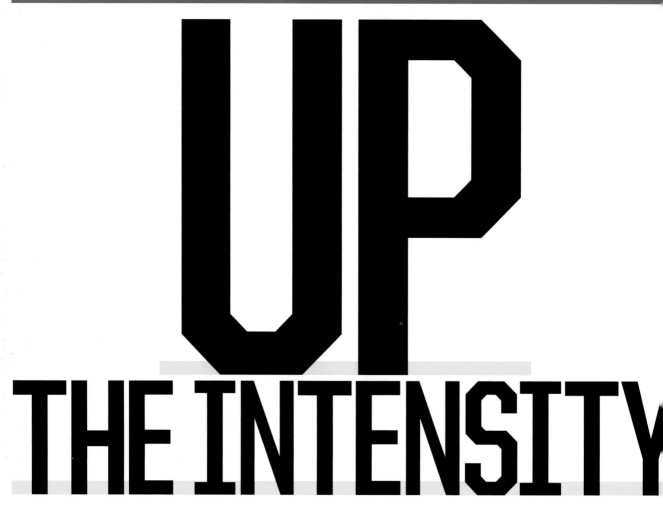

UP THE INTENSITY

In our Ultimate Starter's Guide (Chapter 1), we present you with a plan for building a foundation of muscle that's guaranteed to deliver results for as long as you decide to play the iron game. There will come a time in the near future, however, when you'll want to experiment with more advanced methods, or "intensity techniques," as they're often called. These are ways to tweak the traditional set/rep matrix to increase the intensity of an exercise or of an entire workout. If you're a beginner, we recommend completing the eight weeks of our Ultimate Starter's Guide program before launching into any of the intensity techniques listed here. If you've been at this for a while, you've probably already incorporated a few of the more commonly used ones, like supersets and forced reps. Check out some of the others, like rest-pause sets and dropsets, to increase the intensity even more.

We don't recommend employing more than a couple of these techniques in a single workout, as they're very taxing on the muscles and on your central nervous system. Overtraining and injury are real possibilities if you push it too hard with intensity techniques. However, we encourage you to try them all as you progress. You'll probably come to find that some work better for you than others, and that some are better applied to different body parts and exercises. Regardless, you should store each of these techniques in your training arsenal for future use as you continue to work toward your ultimate physique.

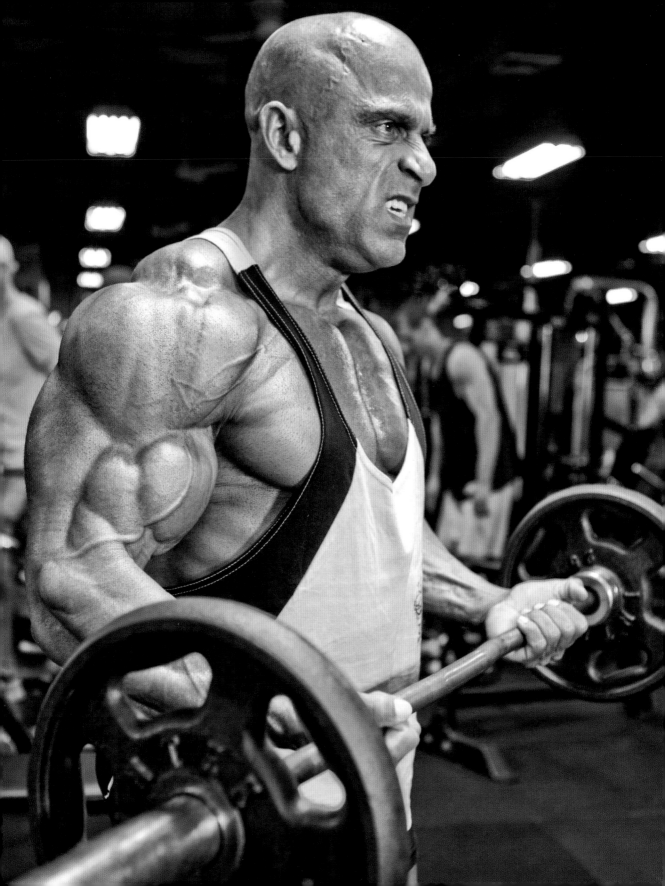

SUPERSET

What it is:
Two sets of different exercises performed back to back with no rest in between. A superset can consist of exercises for different body parts (such as chest and back or quads and shoulders) or the same muscle group (as in two biceps exercises).

Why you should do it:
To burn more calories and get more work done in less time. When supersetting different muscle groups, one body part recovers while the other works, and you can cut rest time in half. When supersetting for the same muscle group, you can thoroughly exhaust it, which is great for bringing up a weak area. New research has found that you burn about 35% more calories during and after a workout that uses supersets versus standard straight sets.

How to do it:
Opposing muscle groups like chest and back are ideal for supersetting to promote muscular balance. Not that there's anything wrong with pairing, say, shoulders and biceps, but opposites always attract with this technique. When supersetting the same muscle group, it's usually preferred to do the more difficult exercise first.

EXERCISE	SETS	REPS	REST
Barbell Curl	3	10-12	—
SUPERSET WITH			
Lying Triceps Extension	3	10-12	1-2 min.
Dumbbell Overhead Extension	2-3	12-15	—
SUPERSET WITH			
Incline Dumbbell Curl	2-3	12-15	1-2 min.

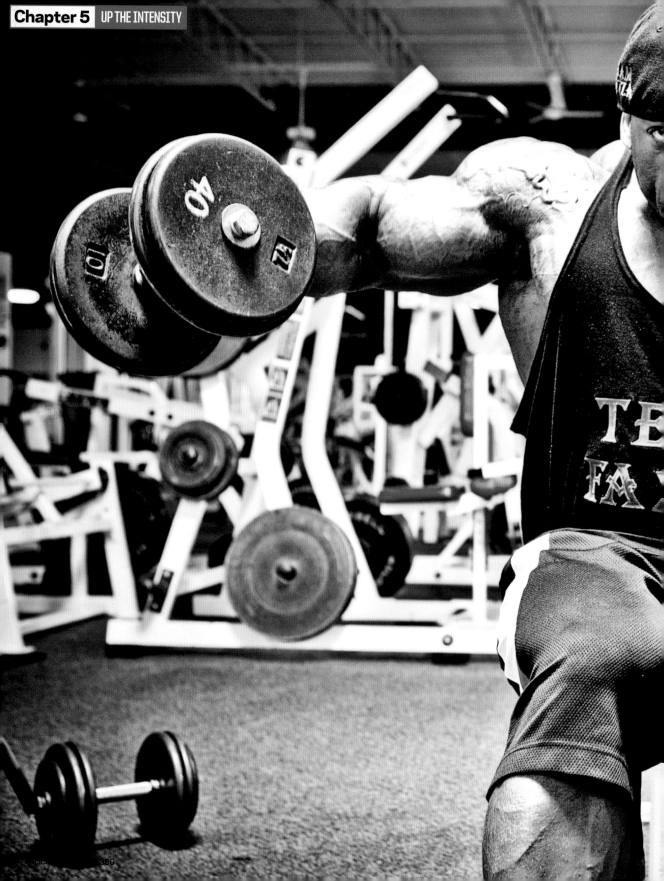

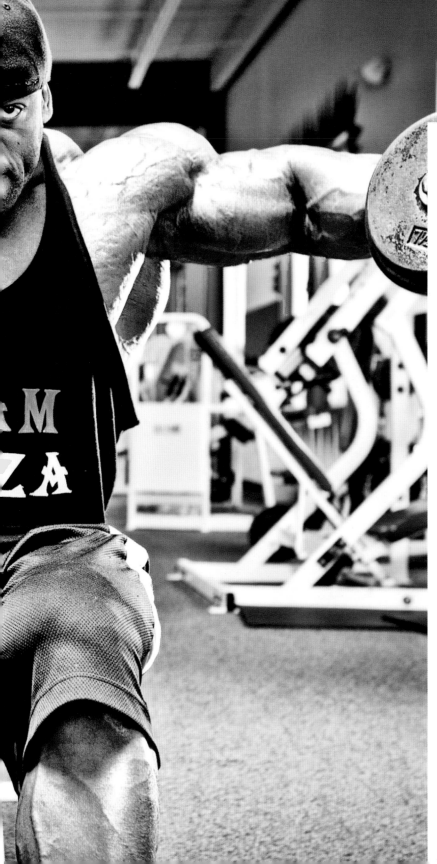

GIANT SET

What it is:
Four or more exercises for one body part performed consecutively without resting between exercises. While a superset can incorporate two different muscle groups, the official definition of a giant set involves only one, whether it be shoulders, chest, back, or legs.

Why you should do it:
To significantly increase volume and intensity for a single body part in the shortest amount of time possible. A giant set is one of the most aggressive ways to attack a weak area in your physique, since you're not only ramping up intensity but hitting the muscle group from a multitude of angles as well.

How to do it:
As with supersetting a single body part, when choosing exercises and a sequence for a giant set, it's best to go from heaviest to lightest—in other words, the exercise that allows you to lift the most weight should be done first, then descend from there (unless you're purposely pre-exhausting to bring up a particular body part). Reason being, you want to maximize the amount of weight lifted through the entire giant set, and if isolation exercises are performed before compound moves, you'll have to go much lighter on the latter. Be careful not to overtrain with this technique. Giant sets are inherently high volume, as every set is multiplied by at least four.

SAMPLE GIANT SET SHOULDER ROUTINE

EXERCISE	SETS	REPS
Seated Overhead Dumbbell Press	3-4	8-10
GIANT SET WITH		
Dumbbell Upright Row	3-4	8-10
GIANT SET WITH		
Dumbbell Lateral Raise	3-4	10-12
GIANT SET WITH		
Dumbbell Bentover Lateral Raise	3-4	10-12

Note: Using dumbbells is a great way to not lose your "station" at the gym as you move from one exercise to the next.

DROPSET

What it is:
A set where, after reaching failure with the initial load, the weight is immediately decreased and reps are performed to failure once again. The set is either finished at this point or multiple dropsets are performed, where the weight is decreased further and failure is reached each time.

Why you should do it:
Dropsets allow you to take your muscles past failure on a given exercise and extend a set without resting, which increases the exhaustion in that muscle group for better gains in size and definition. If you have a weak body part that could use some extra attention, dropsets are ideal.

How to do it:
Dropping the right amount of weight is key, as is exercise selection. If you don't lighten the resistance enough, you'll only be able to do a few more reps, if that; if you drop too much weight, your muscles won't be challenged enough to get the full benefit of the technique. If you failed at, say, 10 reps with the initial weight, you'll want to fail at around that rep count on subsequent dropsets—at 8-10 reps rather than three to five. To achieve this, a good rule of thumb is to decrease the weight 20-30% for each dropset, as research confirms this is the best weight range for optimizing results. For example, if you were using 80-pound dumbbells for bench presses, you would drop to a pair of 55s or 60s, then to a pair of 35s or 40s. The best exercises for dropsets are dumbbell, machine, and cable moves, where weight can be decreased quickly to minimize rest. Picking up a lighter pair of dumbbells only takes seconds. On machines and cables, moving the pin allows quick changes as well.

SAMPLE DROPSET BICEPS ROUTINE

EXERCISE	SETS	REPS	REST
Dumbbell Incline Curl	3*	8-10	2-3 min.
Cable EZ-bar Curl	3*	10-12	2 min.
Preacher Curl	3*	12-15	2 min.

*Perform two dropsets on the last two sets.

PARTIAL REP

What it is:
A technique where reps are performed short of your full range of motion (ROM), typically at the end of a set when strict reps are no longer physically possible due to fatigue, which doesn't allow you to lift the weight past your "sticking point."

Why you should do it:
Because you'd rather not stop to rest, lighten the weight, or end the set just yet. Achieving full ROM is always recommended, but partials, used occasionally, can help you extend a set seamlessly to fatigue your muscle fibers that much more, even if it's just in the bottom or top half of the movement.

How to do it:
The majority of the set is still taken through a full ROM. Using biceps curls as an example, let's say you choose a weight you can do for 10 strict reps. After your 10th rep, when you've reached failure and are unable to move the bar past a certain point, simply do reps where you're lifting the weight as far up as possible.

SAMPLE PARTIAL-REPS LEGS ROUTINE

EXERCISE	SETS	REPS	REST
Squat	4	8-10*	2 min.
Leg Press	3	10-12*	2 min.
Leg Extension	3	12-15*	1-2 min.
Leg Curl	3	12-15*	1-2 min.

Perform partial reps at the end of your last one to two sets after reaching failure on full ROM reps. Do partials until you can no longer budge the weight.

FORCED REP

SAMPLE FORCED-REPS SHOULDER WORKOUT

EXERCISE	SETS	REPS	REST
Barbell Overhead Press	4	8*	2-3 min.
Smith Machine Upright Row	3	10-12*	2 min.
Barbell Front Raise	3	10-12*	2 min.
Cable Lateral Raise	3	12-15	1-2 min.

Perform 2-4 forced reps on your last two sets.

What it is:
A technique where, after reaching failure on a set, a spotter assists in lifting the weight so that you can get past your sticking point and continue the set.

How to do it:
The key to effective forced-rep training is having a spotter who knows what he is doing. The objective is to get two to four forced reps at the end of a set—not 8-10 For that reason, the spotter shouldn't be helping too much and taking on most of the work. He should make you work hard throughout each and every forced rep, providing just enough assistance to get y past your sticking point. That said, the sp ter shouldn't be making you work so hard that the reps each take five seconds on the concentric portion.

Why you should do it:
Research confirms that forced reps increase growth hormone (GH) levels more than sets taken only to muscle failure. This anabolic hormone secreted by the pituitary gland plays a key role in muscle and bone growth. GH is also critical for fat burning—studies have shown that athletes using forced reps drop more body fat than those stopping at failure.

REST-PAUSE SET

What it is:
A set where, after reaching failure, you rest a short period of time and continue to failure once again using the same weight. A typical set in this manner consists of one to three rest-pauses.

How to do it:
Pick the weight you'd normally use for a given set, go to failure, rest 15 seconds, then pick the weight back up and rep out again. Repeat one or two more times. The number of reps you'll be able to perform will decrease significantly with each rest-pause, so don't expect to fail at 10 reps, rest 15 seconds, then get another 10. Chances are, you'll only be able to get three to five more reps tops. One way to avoid a big drop-off is to stop a couple reps short of failure on the initial set, which will allow you to get more reps after resting.

SAMPLE REST-PAUSE BACK ROUTINE

EXERCISE	SETS	REPS	REST
Pullup (or assisted pullup)	3-4	6-8*	2-3 min
Seated Cable Row	3	10-12*	2 min.
Lat Pulldown	3	12*	1-2 min

Perform 2-3 rest-pauses on the last one or two sets.

Why you should do it:
Like dropsets, rest-pauses allow you to take a set of a given exercise past the point of muscle failure, which can lead to gains in m cle size, strength, and shape. But in this case, the short rest peri allows you to stick with the same weight instead of going lighter. a result, what once was a set of 10 reps with 100 pounds becom a set of 15-20 reps with 100 pounds by way of rest-pauses, so more total work has been performed.

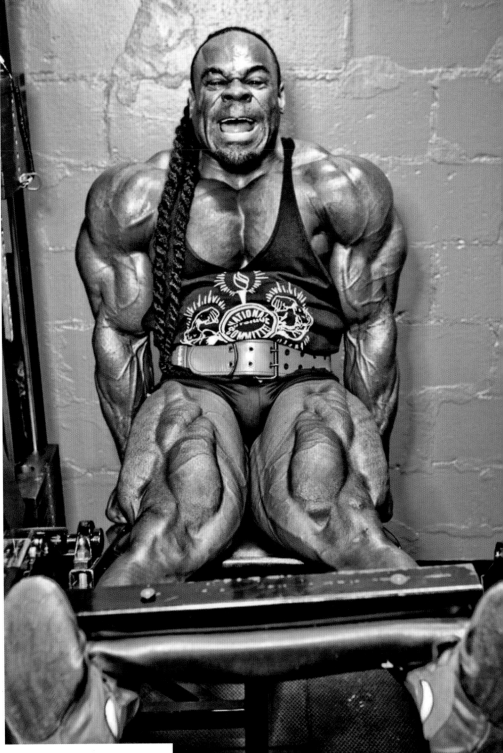

NEGATIVES

What they are:

An advanced method where, with the help of a spotter, only the eccentric (negative) portion of each rep is performed—and at a very slow pace. Traditionally, strength athletes have performed negatives as standalone sets, but this technique can also be used at the end of a regular set to train the muscles past failure.

Why you should do them:

Negatives provide a unique shock to your muscles and are very effective at increasing strength as well as muscle growth. Most people disregard the eccentric portion of the rep, thinking that the muscle is only working when you're lifting the weight, not lowering it. Not true. Resisting the weight on the negative is a crucial aspect of strength and is actually the part of the movement most closely associated with muscle soreness in the days following a workout. And that soreness equates to increases in muscle size and strength.

How to do them:

The specifics of how to do negatives is crucial. First, you'll need a dependable spotter. After reaching failure on a set doing regular reps, you'll do two to three negatives in this manner: your spotter will help you lift the weight through the positive portion of the rep. Then, for the negative, you'll do all the work, lowering the weight slowly for a count of three to five seconds. The spotter will again do the positive, and so on. But even though you'll be lowering the weight on your own, your spotter will need to be highly attentive while you do so in case your muscles give out and you can no longer resist the weight.

SAMPLE NEGATIVES CHEST ROUTINE

EXERCISE	SETS	REPS	REST
Barbell Bench Press	4	8*	2-3 min.
Barbell Incline Press	3-4	10-12*	2 min.
Flat-bench Dumbbell Flye	3	12-15*	1-2 min.

*Do 2-3 negatives on the last two sets.

RAGE WITH THE MACHINES

It's funny how the pendulum swings. In the early days of bodybuilding, serious lifters scoffed at machines, favoring free weights because they provided more functional results and more accurate measures of strength. Then the explosion of Nautilus equipment started people questioning them. And since machines made for better isolation and, in some cases, safer training, it seemed that cables, cams, and levers might be superior bodybuilding tools. Nowadays, any intelligent lifter will make use of both kinds of equipment whenever possible. But if he's already built a good base of strength with free weights, has years of heavy lifting under his weight belt, or is coming back from an injury, he may want to leave the barbell alone. And we've got a machine-based program that works just as well.

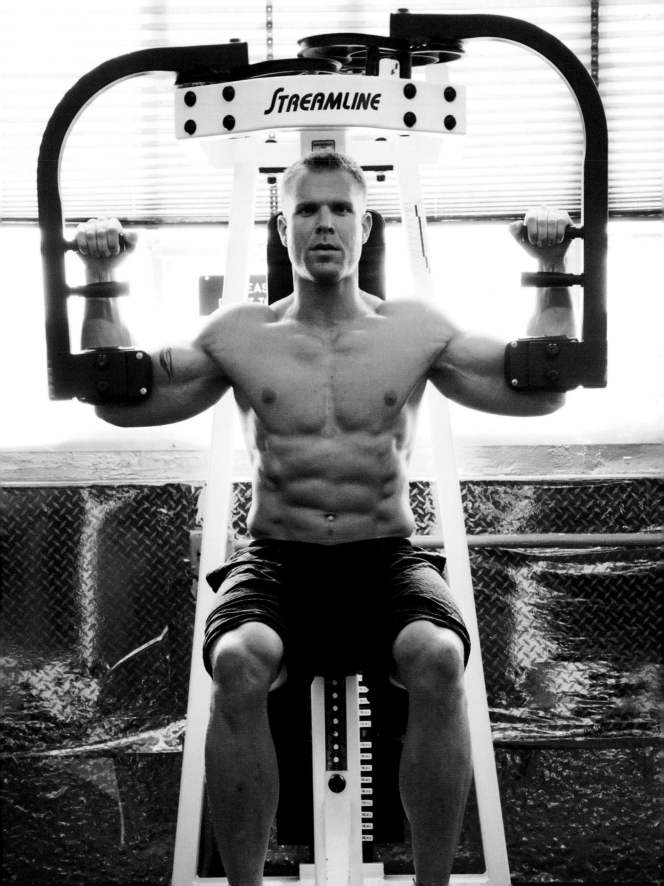

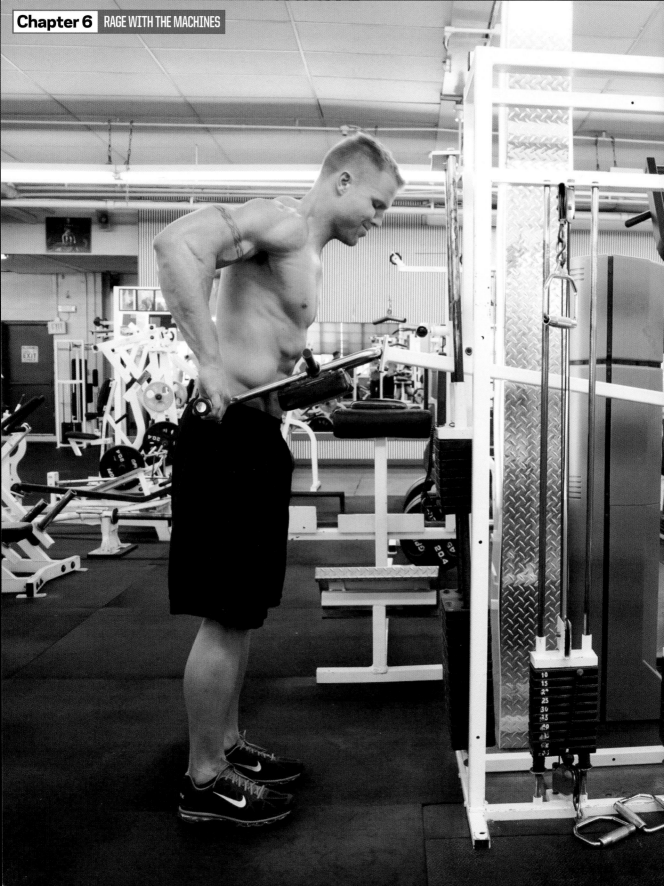

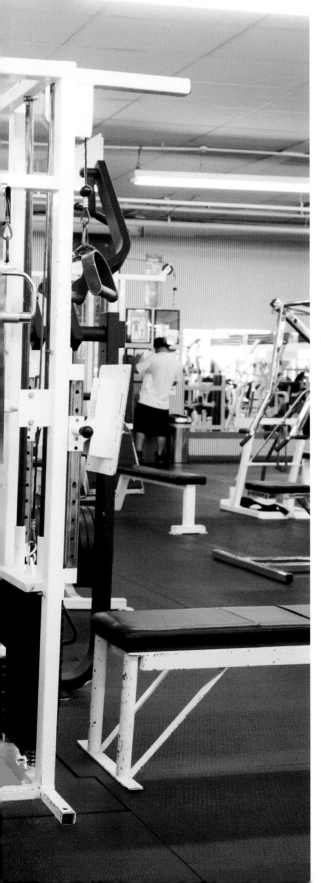

WHAT'S THERE TO RAGE AGAINST?

Look, we love barbells and dumbbells. In fact, *Muscle & Fitness* has done more to popularize them than any other magazine over the years. If you're a young lifter who wants to put on size, get yourself to the squat rack. But older guys who've logged thousands of hours training heavy need a break. Their joints can't handle the strain and would benefit from more isolated movements. Besides, sometimes your body just needs a new stimulus to grow. If you've been benching forever and your chest is still flat, it might be time to hammer it with some pec deck flyes, so your pecs can really be stretched and squeezed with some concentrated time under tension.

While we designed this program to be user-friendly to a longtime reader with some wear and tear, we're not assuming this guy is some softy who's lost the heart to train hard. You're likely to find that our routine is as hardcore as any you've done. We're compensating for the lack of total-body tension you get from free weights with a bevy of intensity techniques—partial reps, rest/pause, and drop-sets—so you can wring out all the effort your muscles have to give while your joints stay protected. The importance of hard work is a concept about which there's never been a back-and-forth debate.

NO PAIN, MORE GAIN
How our machine program will keep you off the DL

>No heavy weights on your back. Instead of squatting or leg pressing on a 45-degree angle and putting your lower back at risk, you'll do leg presses upright.

>No shearing forces on the knees. The knee joint is most unstable when bent 90 degrees. The leg extensions we prescribe will have you stopping short of that, which also keeps high tension on your quads.

>No pressing. You'll work the chest with flye motions that better isolate the pecs and take rotator cuff strain out of the equation.

>Active stretching. Since your knees are held down by the pad, the top position of a lat pull-down stretches the lats and helps unload the spine.

>Heavier isolated training. Lateral raises isolate the delts better than pressing movements, but you can't use heavy weights with them. We've made use of the machine upright row to allow heavier loading without shoulder strain while still focusing on full delt activation.

>Three-day split. By working fewer body parts in a single session, you'll keep the overall stress of your training down and provide more time for recovery.

DIRECTIONS
SPLIT: Perform each workout (Chest/Triceps, Back/Shoulders/Biceps, Legs) once or twice per week. Space rest days as needed.
HOW TO DO IT: Complete two warm-up sets of 20, then do two normal work sets of 12–15 reps. Next, do three sets of 8–10 reps, with each done differently. On the first of these sets, select a weight that causes failure in the 8–10 range and then finish with a few partial reps (go through only the first few inches of the range of motion). On the second set, use a rest/pause. You'll complete your 8–10 reps to failure, rest a few seconds, and then try to force out a few more reps. In the final set, complete 8–10 reps and then do a dropset: reduce the load by 10% and force out a few more reps. Rest 90 seconds to two minutes between all sets.

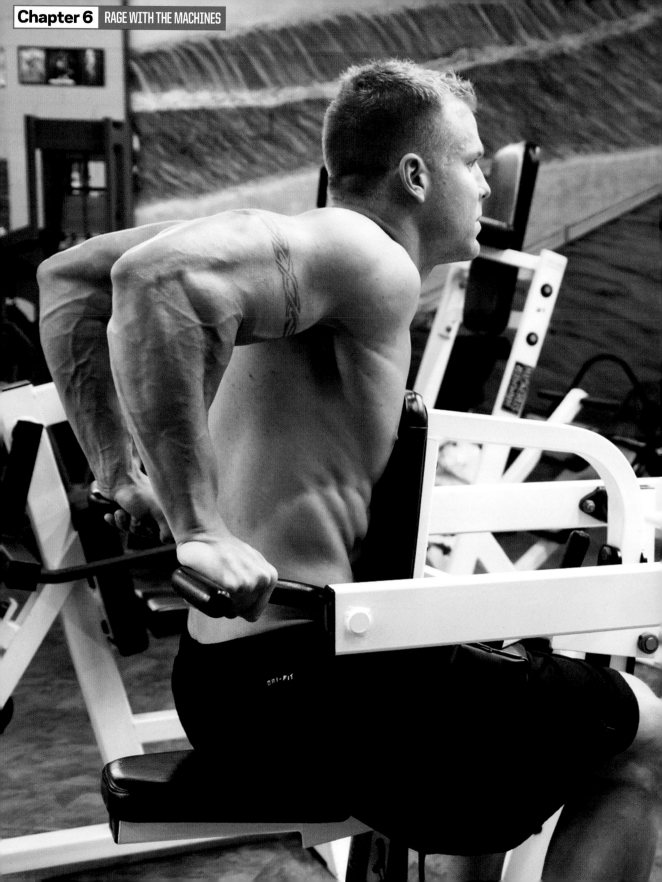

CHEST + TRICEPS

1
Pec-Deck Flye
With your upper arms parallel to the floor and elbows against the pads, squeeze your pecs and bring the handles in front of your chest. Allow your pecs to stretch at the end of the negative portion of each rep.

2
Close-Grip Machine Dip
Sit at a machine dip station and grab the close-grip handles. Press them down and then allow them to come up until your upper arms are parallel to the floor.

3
Crunch
Lie on the floor and cross your arms over your chest. Tuck your chin to your chest and raise your torso until your shoulder blades are off the floor. You can skip the warmup sets here and use weight plates or dumbbells for extra resistance.

4
Back Extension
Climb onto a back extension apparatus and secure your feet. The crease of your hips should be even with the pad edge. Bend forward at the hips until you feel your lower back is about to lose its arch, then use your glutes to extend your hips. Come up until your body forms a straight line.

BACK + SHOULDERS + BICEPS

1
Lat Pulldown
Use a lat pulldown station and secure your knees under the pad. Grab the handle with a grip outside shoulder width and pull it down to your collarbone.

2
Machine Wide-Grip Upright Row
Stand at an upright row machine (a Nautilus bench press machine may work as well if you straddle the bench) and grab the handles with an outside-shoulder-width grip. Squeeze your shoulder blades together as you raise the handles until your upper arms are parallel to the floor.

3
Machine Curl
Use a seated biceps curl machine and rest your triceps against the pad. Curl the weight up until your biceps are fully flexed.

LEGS

1 Upright Leg Press
Sit at a leg press station that allows your torso to stay as vertical as possible. Set your feet against the foot plate at shoulder width and allow your knees to bend to 90 degrees as you breathe in. Press the plate away.

2 Partial Leg Extension
Set up at a leg extension machine and extend your knees until they're fully locked out. Bend your knees to lower the weight but stop three quarters away from a 90-degree knee bend. Keep tension on your quads.

3 Seated Leg Curl
Use a seated leg curl machine and make sure the axis of rotation lines up with your knees. Bend your knees as far as you can against the resistance.

4 Calf Raise on Leg Press Machine
Sit at a leg press machine and place your feet on the foot plate inside shoulder width. Keeping your knees straight, allow your ankles to flex so you feel a stretch in your calves and then contract your calves and drive your toes into the plate to push the weight back.

5 Seated Calf Raise
Sit at a seated calf raise machine and secure your knees under the pad. Lower your heels to the floor until you feel a stretch in your calves and then drive your toes into the plate and raise your heels as high as you can.

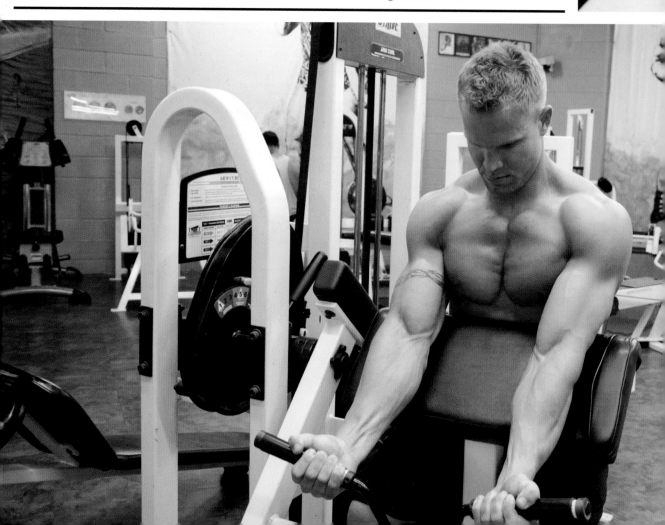

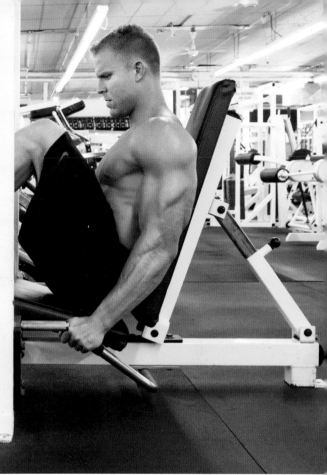

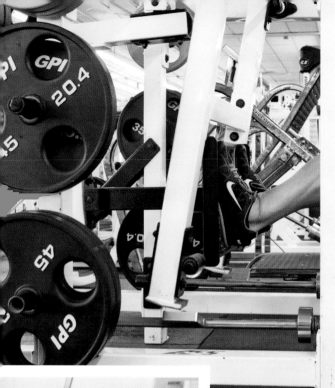

STAVE OFF INJURIES
Keep the injury bug at bay in four simple steps

1
Get an adequate warmup.
Do a general warmup on a cardio machine of your choice for 5–10 minutes, then a specific warmup to send blood to the joints getting the most work. For example: Do two sets of 20 arm circles with five-pound plates on upper-body days, and two or three sets of 15 body-weight squats on lower-body days.

2
No cheating.
If you're twisting into odd positions and squirming to get the weight up (like having to come out of your seat on the preacher curl machine), you're going too heavy.

3
Use deload weeks.

Once every four to six weeks, you need to back away from heavy weights to allow time for recovery and growth.

4
Use recovery workouts.

Don't completely lay off of body parts worked on the previous day. After a big chest workout, it pays to do a few sets of pushups the next day, or some body-weight walking lunges the day after a leg workout. You'll send blood and nutrients to the areas that need them most, help flush away soreness, and speed growth and recovery.

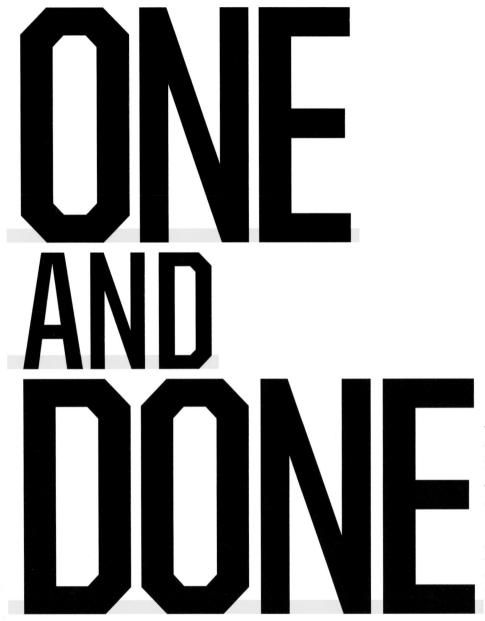

ONE AND DONE

Business, vacation, or holiday travels throug out the year will likely take you somewhere withou a gym or the kind of equipment you're used to. Wheth it's a relative's garage scattered with a few relics of a long-abandoned fitness regimen or a dingy hotel roo more akin to a prison cell, th only thing that can stop you from training hard is your own lack of imagination. We gathered some of the most creative trainers we know a had them lay out one-imple ment workouts. So whether you have a set of dumbbells a lone kettlebell, a rusty old weight plate, or just a chair and the floor, you've got mo than enough to get 'er done

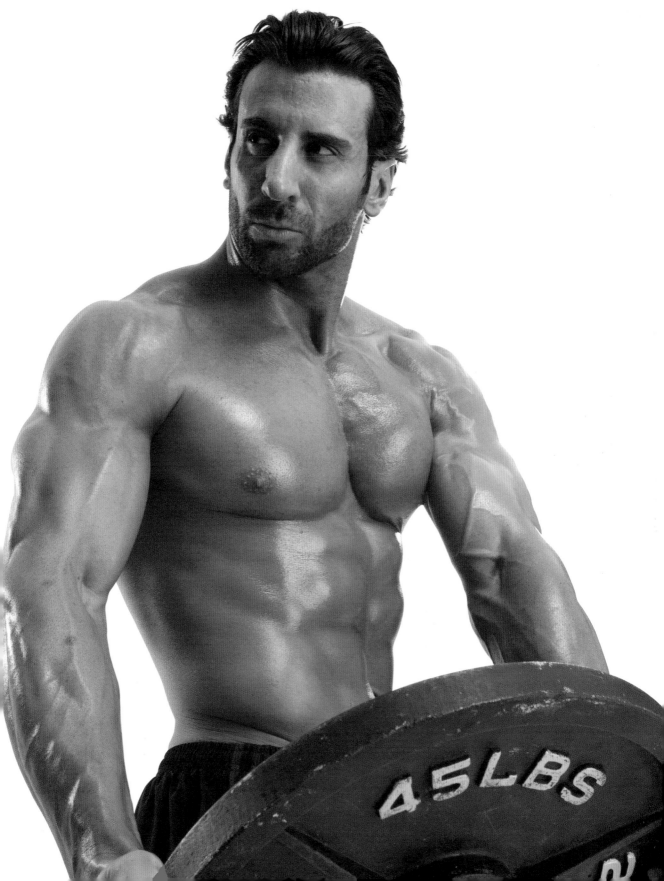

FLOOR

Somehow, you don't have a single piece of equipment—not a band or an old weight in sight. Well, you're not off the hook. You can train with nothing but your body weight—as long as you have a floor under your feet, you're good to go. This regimen from Jon Hinds, owner of the Monkey Bar Gym franchise, will get you by with nothing. (Well, nothing except a deck of cards and something to hang from, and if you don't have those, improvise.)

THE WORKOUT

Grab a deck of cards. A different exercise is assigned to each suit: Hearts are scorpion pushups; diamonds are pullups; spades are a split squat (with rear foot elevated, as shown in the chair workout); and clubs are a hip bridge (with feet elevated, as seen in the chair workout). The value of the card is the number of reps you'll perform. Jacks are 11, queens 12, and so on up. Turn over three cards at a time. Do the reps for the first two cards, and if the third card is of the same suit as the second, add that to the rep count and turn over another card. If that fourth card is also of the same suit, add that as well. Keep going until you get to a different suit. If the third card is a different suit, simply count it in the next three-card turn. For instance, if you pull a five of hearts, a nine of diamonds, and a two of spades, you'd do five scorpion pushups and nine pullups (or as many as you can, resting until you get to nine). You'll count the spades in the next turn. If the third card had been a four of diamonds, you'd have added it to the pull-up reps and then flipped again to see if you got another diamonds card. (If not, you'd have done 13 total reps of pullups and moved on.) Continue this process until you've completed the deck.

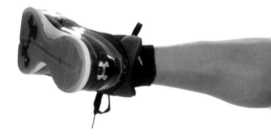

SCORPION PUSHUP

Perform a pushup, but as you lower your body raise your left leg behind your hips and to the right side. It will look like a scorpion's tail. As you push up, return your leg to the floor. Repeat on the opposite side. That's one rep.

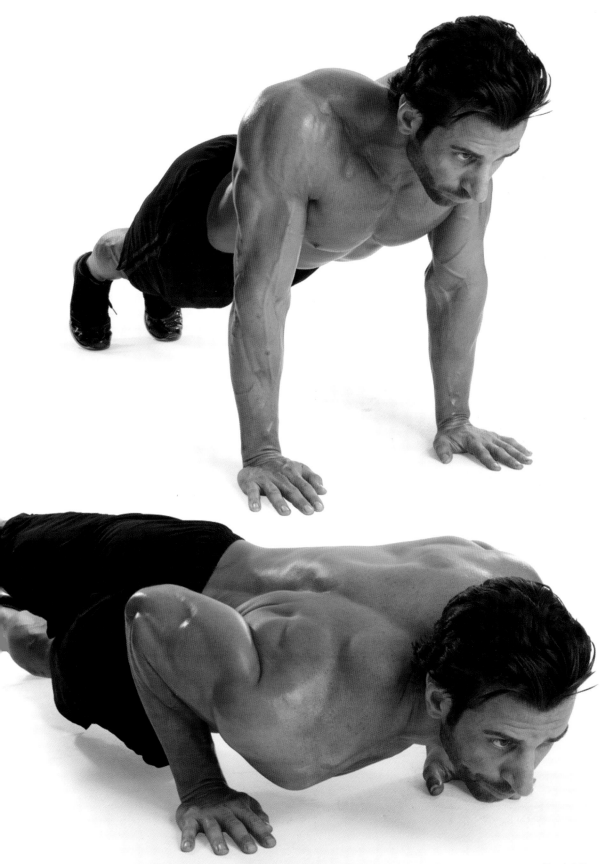

KETTLEBELL

Your mom thought the kettlebell at the yard sale was cute, so she's been using it as a doorstop. You know its true potential. Follow this routine by Marc Bartley, also a certified kettlebell instructor. It'll work for any weight 'bell.

THE WORKOUT

Alternate between two-hand kettlebell swings and one-arm snatches, spending a minute performing reps with each. Pace yourself. The goal is to keep going for 20 minutes.

Minute 1:
Righthand Snatch
Minute 2:
Two-hand Swing
Minute 3:
Lefthand Snatch
Minute 4:
Two-hand Swing
Repeat for 20 min.

If you have a very heavy kettlebell, you can switch hands after 30 seconds. The workout would then look like this.
Minute 1:
Righthand Snatch, 30 sec.
Lefthand Snatch, 30 sec.
Minute 2:
Two-hand Swing
And so on

ONE-ARM SNAT
Hold the kettlebe front of you at ar length, palm faci you. Bend your h back until the we rests on the floo Extend your hips and knees explo- sively, shrugging your shoulder an coming up on the balls of your feet you pull the weig up. Let the mom tum help carry it straight overhea Lower the weigh your shoulder ar then the floor.

TWO-HAND SWING
Stand with feet shoulder width, holding the kettlebell with both hands. Bend the hips so the weight hangs between your legs. Explosively extend your hips and knees to swing the weight up until your arms are parallel to the floor. Let the momentum carry the bell back down and use your stretch reflex to begin the next rep.

45-POUND PLATE

Got a spare 45-pound weight plate lying around? Here's what you can do with it besides playing Frisbee, according to Keith Scott, a strength coach and physical therapist based in Medford, NJ.

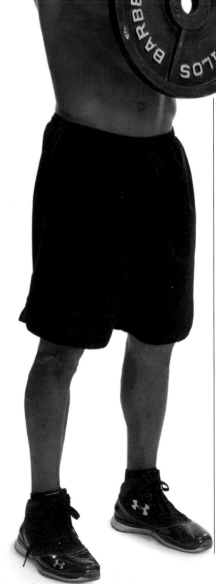

UPRIGHT ROW

THE WORKOUT

Do the exercise pairs (marked "A" and "B") as supersets (try not to rest at all in between them). To use lighter plates, such as 25s, just adjust your tempo—perform the exercises more explosively and power through them, or go slower to test your endurance.

1A PLATE SQUAT
SETS: 3
REPS: 8-12
Hold the plate with both hands and extend your arms in front of you (keep them straight or only slightly bent). Squat down as far as you can and then explode back up to starting position. Keep your core tight.

1B PLATE CURL/ PRESS/SQUAT
SETS: 3
REPS: 8-12
Hold the plate flat, resting it on your thighs. Curl the weight up to your face slowly, and then press the plate over your head. Then, while holding the plate over your head, perform a squat.

2A RUSSIAN TWIST
SETS: 3
REPS: 8-12
(EACH SIDE)
Sit on the floor, knees bent, holding a plate. Lean back, then move the plate from side to side, bringing it as close as you can to the floor on each side.

2B OVERHEAD TRICEPS EXTENSION
SETS: 3
REPS: 8-12
Hold the plate with both hands overhead. Start with your arms bent and the plate resting behind your head. Slowly extend your elbows to raise the plate, keeping your elbows pointed forward.

3A REVERSE CHOP
SETS: 3
REPS: 12-15
(EACH SIDE)
Hold the plate in both hands by your right hip. Bring the plate up and across your body toward your head in a reverse chopping motion.

3B SUITCASE DEADLIFT
SETS: 3
REPS: 8-12
(EACH SIDE)
Hold the plate in one hand at your side; squat to touch it to the floor.

4A SHOULDER RAISE W/HOLD
SETS: 3
REPS: 8-12
Hold the plate resting on your thighs. Keeping your arms as straight as you can, slowly raise the plate to face level and hold it for 10–15 seconds.

4B UPRIGHT ROW
SETS: 3
REPS: 12-15
Hold the top edge of the plate with both hands so the hole is facing your body. Row the plate upward until your hands and the plate reach your chin.

5A PLATE PUSHUP
SETS: 3
REPS: 15-25
Do pushups with the plate on your back, keeping it stable as possible.

5B PLATE PRESS W/ EXTENSION
SETS: 3
REPS: 10-12
Lie on your back while holding the plate on your chest. Press it up, then bend your elbows to lower it to your forehead. Extend your elbows and return the weight to your chest.

DUMBBELLS

mewhere in your uncle's shed lies a pair
dumbbells. Maybe they're selectorized,
e Powerblocks or the Bowflex SelectTech
t, which would give you more options,
t more than likely they're a pair of 35s.
matter. Here's what you do with them,
prescribed by Marc Bartley, a strength
ach in Columbia, SC.

E WORKOUT

e the dumbbells probably
't heavy, your best bet is to
struct a 30- to 45-minute
ure session working the
le body. Lifting with a slow-
nore deliberate tempo will
lighter weights feel heavier,
lenge your endurance, and
ease your concentration on
h rep. Aim for every set to
a minute and, depending on
load, go for 12–20 reps. (If
have a selectorized dumb-
set, you can go heavier for

lower reps if you like.)
   Pick five exercises from
the following lists of upper-
body, ab, and lower-body
moves. Your workout will consist of 15 total exercises. Do
one move from each category
in sequence—that's one round.
Complete five total rounds,
resting 15–30 seconds be-
tween rounds by walking around
the room. See the sample workout below for some ideas of
how to construct it.

RUSSIAN TWIST

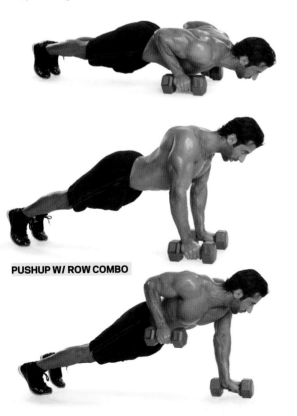

PUSHUP W/ ROW COMBO

EXERCISE OPTIONS
LOWER BODY
Dumbbell Lunge
Front Squat
Clean
Snatch
Overhead Squat
Squat Thrust w/
Dumbbells in Hands
Squat w/Lateral-
Raise Combo
Romanian Deadlift
Abs
Straight-leg Situp
w/Arms Raised Over-
head (no dumbbells
necessary)
Russian Twist
Side Bend
Side Plank w/
Lateral Raise
Crunch w/Dumbbells
Modified Turkish
Get-up

UPPER BODY
Floor Press
Flye on Floor
Pushup w/

Row Combo
Pullover on Floor
Row from Floor
Rolling Triceps
Extension
Overhead Triceps
Extension
Walking Overhead
Dumbbell Hold
Bentover Lateral
Raise
Front or Lateral Raise

SAMPLE DUMB-BELL WORKOUT
ROUND 1
1 Dumbbell Lunge
2 Straight-leg Situp
w/Arms Raised
Overhead
3 Flye on Floor
(Lower your arms un-
til your triceps touch
the floor.)
4 Rest
ROUND 2
1 Romanian Deadlift
2 Modified Turkish
Get-up
3 Pushup w/

Row Combo
4 Rest
ROUND 3
1 Overhead Squat
2 Russian Twist
3 Row from Floor
(Lower the weight
until it makes a dead
stop on the floor.)
4 Rest
ROUND 4
1 Clean
2 Side Bend
3 Rolling Triceps
Extension
4 Rest
ROUND 5
1 One-arm Snatch
2 Crunch w/
Dumbbells
3 Floor Press
(Lie on your back on
the floor and lower
dumbbells as in a
bench press. When
your triceps touch
the floor, press up.)
4 Rest

CHAIR

If you can sit down, you can train. Try this tough chair routine from Keith Scott.

THE WORKOUT

Perform the pairs as supersets.

1A FEET-ELEVATED PUSHUP
SETS: 4
REPS: 15-25
Rest your feet on the chair and do pushups.

1B FEET-ELEVATED UP/DOWN PLANK
SETS: 4
REPS: REPEAT FOR 30-45 SECONDS
Start from the up position of a pushup with your feet on the chair. Move into a plank with forearms flat on the floor, then back to the pushup.

2A STEP-UP
SETS: 3
REPS: 12-15 (EACH LEG)
Step up onto the chair with one foot.

2B SPLIT SQUAT
SETS: 3
REPS: 12-15 (EACH LEG)
With your back to the chair, place the top of one foot on it. Bend the front leg to 90 degrees.

3A FEET-ELEVATED BODY SAW
SETS: 3
REPS: 15-20
Get into a plank with your feet on the chair and rock your body forward so your face moves toward your hands. Push yourself back.

3B FEET-ELEVATED DYNAMIC SIDE PLANK
SETS: 3
REPS: 15-20 (EACH SIDE)
Lie on your side with your feet on a chair and your weight on your forearm. Bridge your hips until your body is straight; lower back down.

4A DOUBLE CHAIR DIP
SETS: 3
REPS: 8-12
Place your palms on the seats of two chairs. Stretch your legs out in front of you, lower yourself until your upper arms are parallel to the floor, then press yourself back up.

4B AROUND-THE-WORLD PLANK
SETS: 3
REPS: 5-10 (EACH SIDE)
In pushup position with your feet on a chair, walk your hands to one side and then the other.

5A SINGLE-LEG HIP BRIDGE
SETS: 3
REPS: 20-25 (EACH LEG)
Rest one foot on a chair and bridge your hips up until your body forms a straight line.

5B PISTOL SQUAT
SETS: 3
REPS: 8-12 (EACH LEG)
Secure the chair and stand on top of it with one leg. Bend your knee and squat down until your free foot touches the floor. Come back up.

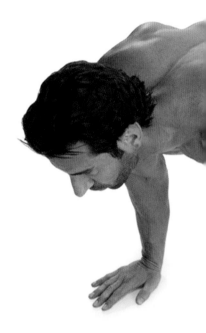

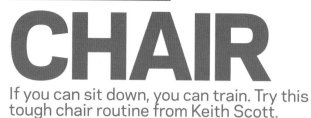

FEET-ELEVATED DYNAMIC SIDE PLANK

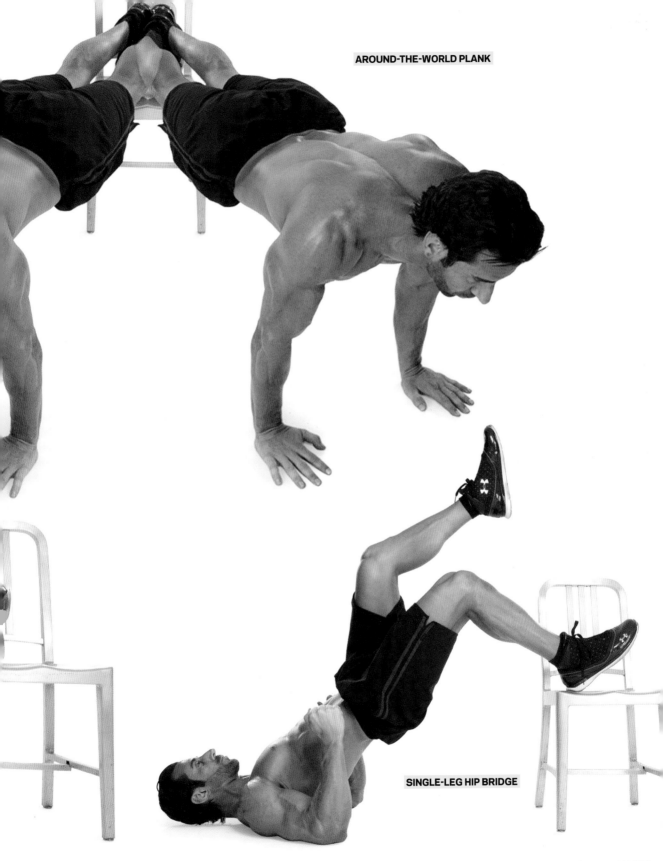

AROUND-THE-WORLD PLANK

SINGLE-LEG HIP BRIDGE

Chapter 8

DON'T JUST GET BIG. BUILD SIZE, STRENGTH, AND ATHLETIC POWER WITH RUSSIA'S GREATEST EXPORT: THE KETTLEBELL.
BY STEVE COTTER

RING

THE

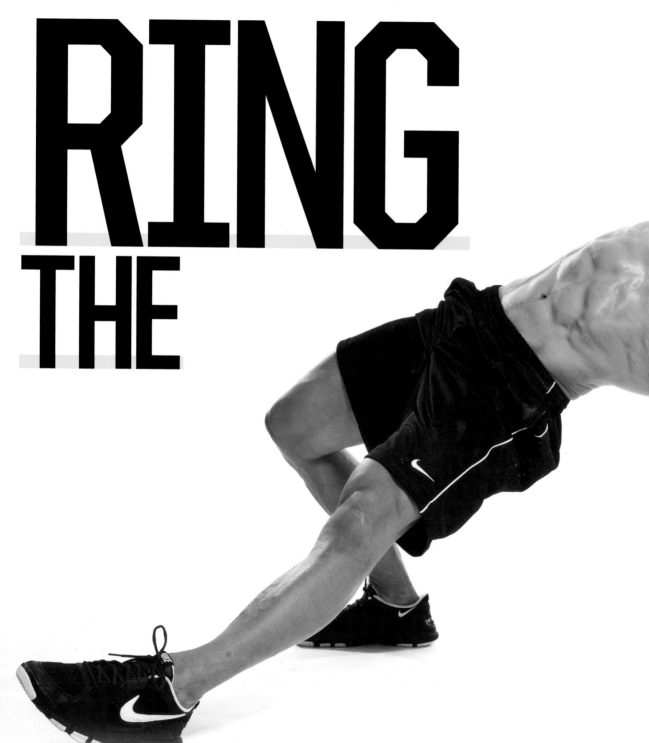

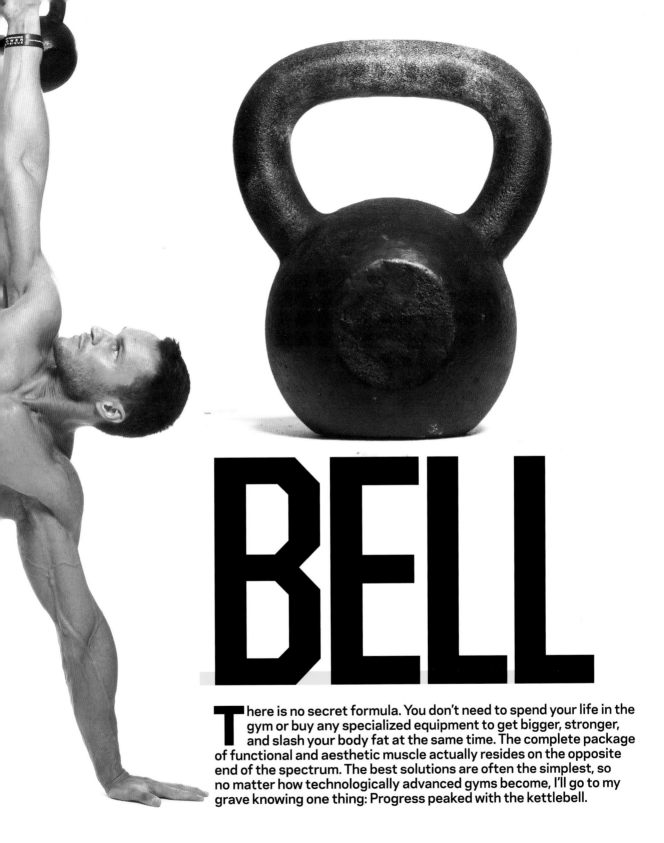

BELL

There is no secret formula. You don't need to spend your life in the gym or buy any specialized equipment to get bigger, stronger, and slash your body fat at the same time. The complete package of functional and aesthetic muscle actually resides on the opposite end of the spectrum. The best solutions are often the simplest, so no matter how technologically advanced gyms become, I'll go to my grave knowing one thing: Progress peaked with the kettlebell.

WITH

a history that dates back to 18th-century Russia, kettlebells lead the pack of old-school training implements that have hit the scene in recent years, with widespread acceptance in the United States occurring over the past decade. The U.S. Navy SEALs, San Diego Chargers, San Francisco 49ers, and the Texas Rangers are just a few organizations I consult with as the president of the International Kettlebell and Fitness Federation, and all have embraced the methods described here. I train with kettlebells exclusively—no other tool has allowed me to stay lean and muscular at a meager 6% body fat.

Best of all, I never need a gym.

The kettlebell doesn't look like much—it's just a cast-iron ball with a handle—but the asymmetrical displacement of the weight (as opposed to the symmetrical balance of a dumbbell) provides a unique stimulus that most trainees aren't used to.

The program we've provided here will have you training four days a week for six weeks, with one workout for Mondays and Thursdays and another for Tuesdays and Fridays. Swings are one of two movements that you'll do every day of the program. They are metabolically demanding, recruit a large muscle area, and reinforce key athletic movements: hip flexion and extension. The swinging exercises will also elevate your heart rate right from the start, and the short rest times (30–60 seconds between sets) will keep it there. If your gym doesn't have a wide selection of kettlebells, I recommend logging on to *ikff.net* and purchasing the two sets you'll need for this workout: a pair of 35-pound kettlebells and a pair of 45-pounders. You'll also need a 55-pound set for one exercise, but dumbbells work just as well, too. Power exercises like cleans and snatches are included in both sessions and will help you build total-body strength and coordination. They're not the easiest lifts to master and require just as much technique as strength.

The following pages break down the program step by step. Slower total-body movements like the overhead squat, one-leg deadlift, Turkish get-up, windmill, and farmer's hold increase your time under tension, so even though these sessions take only 30–40 minutes to complete, there's enough stimulus here to instigate serious muscle growth. There is no direct ab isolation, but there's enough core work—as well as a challenging cardio component—to help carve out your midsection.

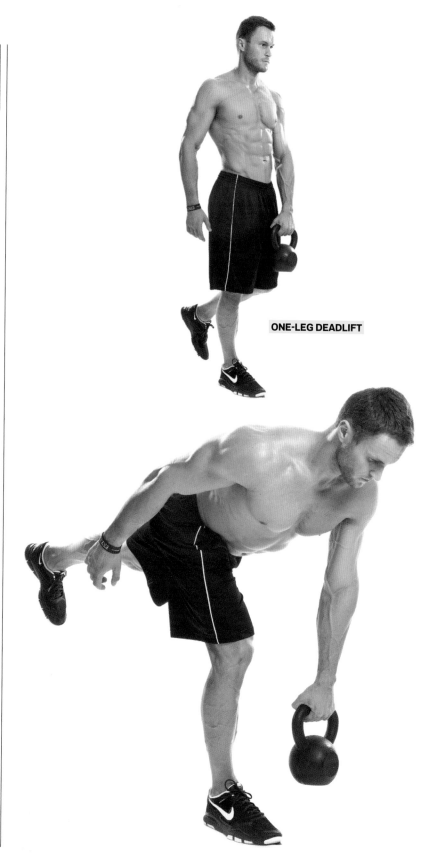

ONE-LEG DEADLIFT

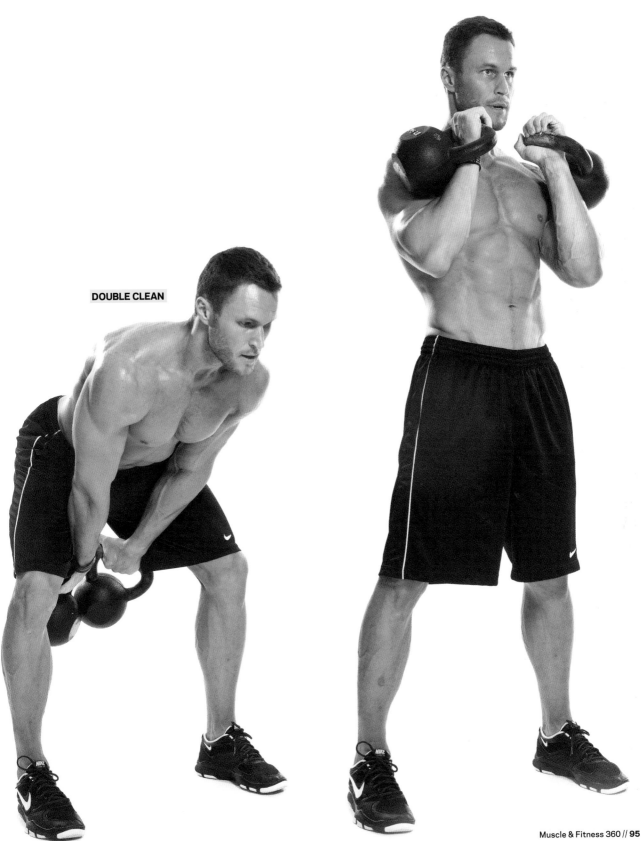

DOUBLE CLEAN

THE WORKOUTS
MONDAY &

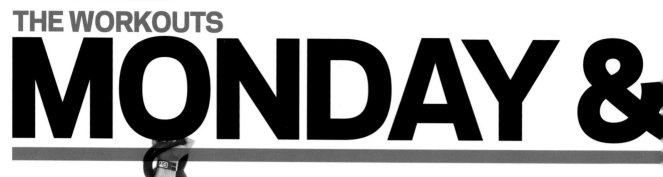

WINDMILL

THURSDAY

TWO-HAND SWING
1x15 with 35 [pounds]; rest 30 seconds before moving to next move

ONE-HAND SWING
1x10 each hand with 35s; rest 30 seconds between each side

ONE-ARM CLEAN AND PUSH PRESS
1x10 each hand with 35s; rest one minute; then do 1x10 with each hand using 45s; rest one minute -before moving on to next move

BOTTOMS-UP CLEAN
2x5 each hand with 45s; rest 30 seconds between sets

WINDMILL
2x5 each hand with 35s; rest 30 seconds between sets

FRONT SQUAT
3x10 with two 35s; rest one minute between sets

HAND-TO-HAND SWING
1x50 with 45s

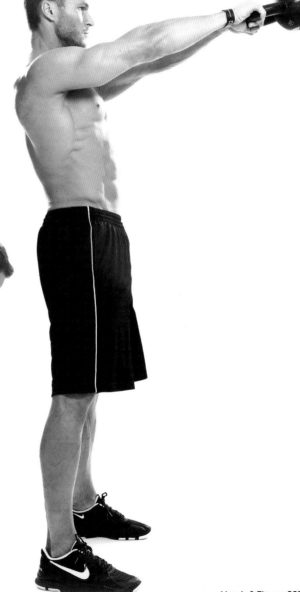

TWO-HAND SWING

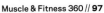

THE WORKOUTS
TUESDAY 8

THE MOVES
Proper execution is dependent on mobility, so be sure to warm up and stretch for 5–10 minutes before beginning the program.

WINDMILL
Clean and press a kettlebell overhead and keep your elbow locked out at all times. Stick your hips out in the direction of the locked-out arm and bend to the opposite side, keeping your core tight. Reach down and touch the floor with your free arm.

SNATCH
Swing one kettlebell back between your legs, then reverse direction to propel the weight toward the ceiling. When the kettlebell reaches eye level, momentarily loosen your grip to slide your hand underneath the kettlebell as it continues to swing overhead. Finish by punching up toward the ceiling and locking out your elbow.

BOTTOMS-UP CLEAN
Perform a one-arm clean, swinging the weight back between your legs and propelling it upward, keeping it close to your body. Finish with the bottom of the kettlebell facing straight up.

TWO-HAND SWING
In a wide stance, hold on to a kettlebell with both hands. Bend your hips and swing the kettlebell backward like you're hiking a football, then explosively extend your hips to swing the weight up to eye level. Allow momentum to keep continuous movement throughout this exercise.

ONE-HAND SWING*
See directions for two-hand swing; perform with one arm.

FRONT SQUAT*
Clean two kettlebells to the rack position. Squat low, leading with your hips and keeping your back in a neutral position. Press your heels into the floor and engage your glutes and hamstrings to return to standing.

HAND-TO-HAND SWING*
Perform a one-arm swing and reach for the weight with your free hand when it comes up to eye level. Quickly release your working hand and grab the weight with your free hand. Alternate hands with each rep.

ONE-ARM CLEAN AND PUSH PRESS*
Perform a one-arm clean to the rack position (your thumb touching your chest and the weight resting on your forearm]. The weight should stay close to your body and the transition should be smooth, meaning the weight doesn't "flop" onto your forearm. Bend your knees, then quickly extend them to press the weight overhead.

DOUBLE CLEAN
Swing two kettlebells back between your legs. Use hip and knee drive and pull from your traps and shoulders to propel the kettlebells upward, keeping them close to your body. Flip your wrists under the kettlebells as they reach your chest. Finish in the rack position, with the weights resting on your forearms and your hands in the middle of your chest.

OVERHEAD SQUAT*
Clean and press two kettlebells overhead. Keeping your elbows locked out and your core muscles tight, squat low to the ground.

ONE-LEG DEADLIFT
Hold a kettlebell in your left hand and let it hang at your side. Bend your left knee and let your left toe rest on the floor. Reach for the ground with the weight and lift your left leg out straight behind you, keeping your back flat. When the kettlebell touches the floor, reverse direction.

ALTERNATING PRESS*
Clean two kettlebells to the rack position. Press the right kettlebell overhead, rotating your hand so your palm faces forward at the finish. Alterna arms until you hit 20 total reps.

FARMER'S HOLD*
Stand up straight holding 53-pou kettlebells or 55-pound dumbbell for one minute. Keep your core tig

TURKISH GET-UP
Lie on the floor with your right knee bent, your right arm raised holding a kettlebell. Stand up, keeping the weight locked out at all times with your eyes on the weight, in this sequence: (1) Shift your weight to you left elbow (not shown); (2) Extend y elbow so that your weight is on you free hand; (3) Press your right foot the floor to extend your hips off the ground; (4) Swing your left foot bac behind you so that your left knee is the floor; (5) Take your free hand of the floor; (6) Keep your abs tight ar stand up. Reverse the entire proce to return to the starting position.

*Exercise Not Shown

FRIDAY

**ND-TO-HAND
ING**
30 with 35s

RKISH GET-UP
5 each side with
s; rest one min-
between sets

UBLE CLEAN
10 with 35s, then
10 with 45s; rest
 minute between
s

**TERNATING
ESS**
10 each side with
s, then 2x5 each
e with 45s; rest
 minute between
s

ERHEAD SQUAT
10 with 35s; rest
 minute between
s

SNATCH
1x10 each hand
with 35s, then 3x10
each hand with 45s,
1x25 each hand
with 35s; rest one
minute between
sets

**ONE-LEG
DEADLIFT**
2x5 each leg with
35s, then 2x5 each
leg with 45s; rest
one minute between
sets

FARMER'S HOLD
2x60 seconds with
55s; rest one min-
ute between sets

STEEL-BELTED STRENGTH

Get outside. For years, we've advocated getting out of the gym and shifting your training to the great outdoors when the weather warms up—and we're not about to change that. Training outside is fun and different, and it's a welcome change of pace after a winter spent inside, but running hills and doing pullups on the monkey bars will take you only so far.

Fitness solutions occasionally come in peculiar forms, and you might just find yours as a result of someone else's bad luck. We're asking you to head down to your local tire store and pick up a pair of worn-out radials or flats. Heavier is better when it comes to used tires, but you don't have to look for any particular make or model, because all you're going to do is take them to the park and use them to get bigger, stronger, and more powerful by dragging and throwing them all over the yard. On the following pages, we'll show you how.

FORWARD DRAG
Hold the handles either behind you or tight to your body in front of you in a comfortable position and walk forward, taking long, powerful strides.

TRAIN HARDER LONGER

Dragging tires will get you in better shape, but in order to understand why, we need to be more specific. In this case, we're referring to something called work capacity—the amount of time you're capable of training at a high enough level to experience significant benefit from the type of exercise you're doing. If you increase your work capacity, your training volume will increase, and you'll get stronger and build muscle at a much faster rate.

Along with recovery methods like contrast showers, massage, ice, and heat, work capacity is the most important piece of your training puzzle in terms of what you need to do to support your actual gym lifting foundation. Adding tire dragging to your regimen will allow you to raise your work capacity in each individual muscle group—which, in turn, will enable you to train for longer periods of time with heavier weight and more sets and reps for each body part.

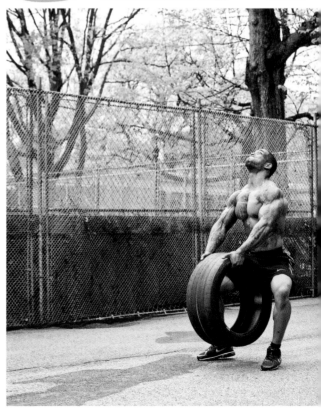

BACKWARD THROW
Stand the tire up and let it sit between your legs. Using both hands, extend your ankles, knees, and hips to throw it as far overhead and behind you as you can.

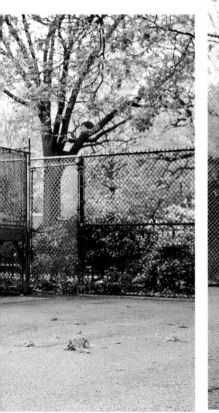

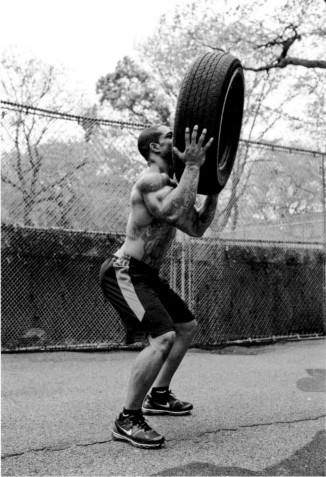

FORWARD THROW
Stand the tire up and let it sit between your legs. Using both hands, extend your ankles, knees, and hips to throw it as far overhead and in front of you as you can.

SIDE THROW

Standing with your target to one side, hold the inside edge of the tire in an overhand grip outside your back leg. Propel the tire directly to your side by rotating as quickly and powerfully as possibly and extending your arms directly toward your target.

ELIMINATE THE NEGATIVE

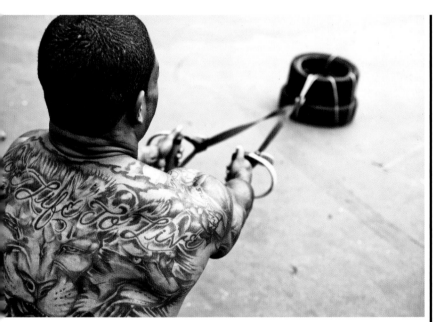

TIRE ROW
Stand facing the tire, with your knees bent and a slight bend at your waist. Back up until your arms are fully extended and there's tension in the straps. Pull the tire as close to you as you can, keeping both hands at the same height as your belly button. Step backward until you're back in the start position and repeat.

Dragging takes away the eccentric—negative—portion of conventional gym movements. To see how this works, let's examine the tire row exercise pictured later in this chapter. All you have to do is step back until all the slack is gone from the straps you're using, then row the tire as far as you can toward you. What you'll notice here is that the tire isn't pulling back. The only resistance you'll encounter is the friction between the tire and the ground. It slides wherever you pull it, but the resistance isn't constant, and comes to an end when you're finished pulling. Moving this way will allow you to improve the work capacity in your lats without beating them up like you do with conventional weight training.

Research has shown that it's the eccentric portion of each lift that does the most tissue damage, so when you remove this part of a movement from the equation, you're not breaking down muscle like you do when training with weights or machines. Instead, you're encouraging blood flow to the area you're working. This causes muscle tissue to repair itself much faster than it otherwise would.

In concentrating solely on the concentric—positive—portion of each move, you'll build work capacity and encourage tissue repair in whatever muscle group you're focused on without the additional negative stress that's so taxing on your joints, ligaments, and tendons. This will enhance the work you're doing in the gym by accelerating the regeneration of the muscle tissue you're trying so hard to grow.

GEOMETRY LESSONS

Targeting specific muscle groups through tire dragging is a matter of angles—and you can train any body part for either power, endurance, or recovery purposes. Just align your body and the strap handles to provide resistance for the muscle you're looking to hit. For example, if you want to focus on your biceps, stand facing the tire, hold the handles in an underhand grip, then adjust your stance and arm angle so that the only way you can move the tire is with a curling motion.

This is where you can be creative, and there's virtually no limit to the moves you can invent. The list we've provided here is a great place to start, but don't stop there. If there's a particular gym exercise you like, figure out how to perform it with your tire and straps and go for it. Want to do leg extensions? Wrap the straps around one ankle, raise your knee in the air so your thigh is parallel to the ground, then use your quads to extend your leg as far as you can. Walk forward and repeat.

We're also throwing in some explosive moves in the form of forward, backward, and side tire throws. The forward and backward throws will improve your explosive power—in addition to working your shoulders, chest, quads, hamstrings, and hips—and the side throws are a highly effective way to work your core rotational strength.

Finally, there's literally nothing better than dragging when it comes to endurance work. Simply grab the handles and start walking, or even running. When you have a tire dragging behind you, you'll feel a definite strain in your hamstrings, abs, and lower back—more so than you would from simply running up a hill. This means you're developing work capacity in your posterior chain—the place you need it most when it comes to building a bigger and stronger lower body. To fry your quads, turn around and drag the tire backward to the line you started from.

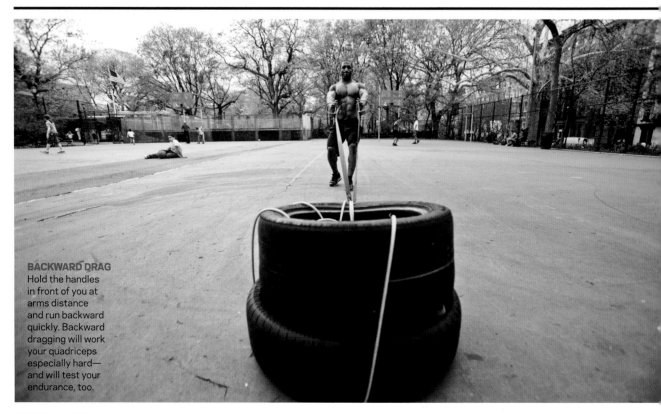

BACKWARD DRAG
Hold the handles in front of you at arms distance and run backward quickly. Backward dragging will work your quadriceps especially hard— and will test your endurance, too.

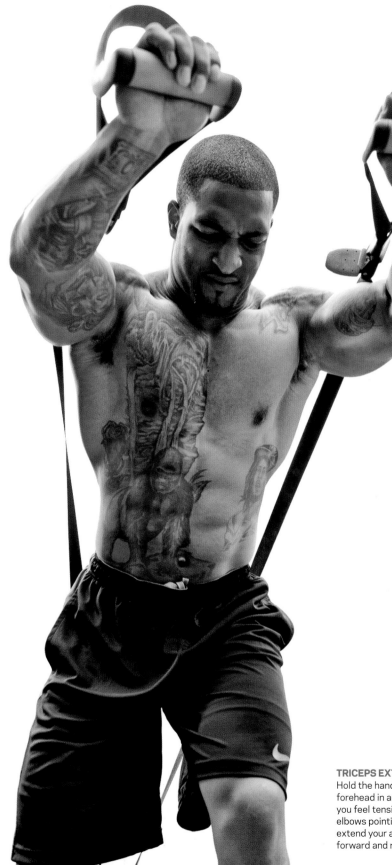

TRICEPS EXTENSION
Hold the handles close together, just over your forehead in an overhand grip. Walk forward until you feel tension in the straps. Keeping your elbows pointing forward, use your triceps to extend your arms in front of you, then step forward and repeat.

THE WORKOUT

Measure a segment of 30-40 yards on grass or pavement. Each segment counts as one trip. When you reach the finish line of a trip, turn around and come back. Rest 30 seconds between trips. Perform the Day 1 workout the day after an intense upper-body workout, and the Day 2 workout the day after you train your legs.

DAY 1

EXERCISE	TRIPS/REPS
Forward Drag	4
Tire Press	4
Triceps Extension	4
Biceps Curl	4
Rear-Delt Flye	4**
Tire Row	4
Forward Drag	6*

DAY 2

EXERCISE	TRIPS/REPS
Forward Drag	4
Forward Throw	8 reps
Backward Throw	8 reps
Side Throw (each side)	8 reps
Backward Drag	4
Pull Through	4**
Forward Drag	8*

*Walk as fast as you can, taking 15 seconds to rest between sets.
**Not pictured.

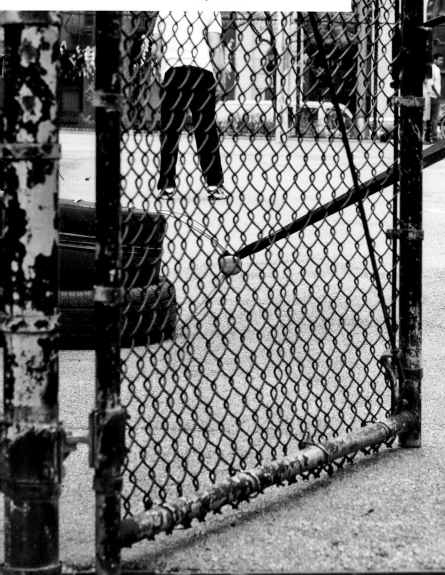

BICEPS C
Stand facing the s
holding the s
handles in an ur
hand grip with
arms extended.
the tire toward
until your hands
as close to your f
delts as possible. S
backward until the
tension in the st
again, and rep

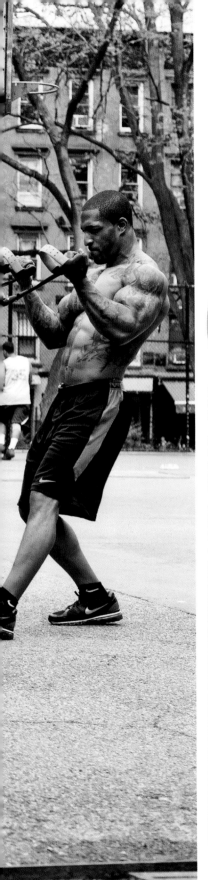

ON THE CHEAP

Procuring a used tire is easy. Just walk into your local tire store or mechanic's garage and ask if you can have one. These places pay to have old tires carted off so taking one is doing the shop a favor.

Once you have a set of tires, you'll need two more things: something to fasten them together, and something you can use to pull them. To bind your tires, stack one on top of the other and use a light chain or an old belt to keep them in place. You'll want something you can attach and detach quickly, so you can add and subtract weight on the fly. If you're dragging your tire across pavement, use a durable object like a coated chain that can withstand the friction without damaging the pavement surface.

From here, attach a set of Jungle Gym XT or TRX suspension straps—or a rope with loops tied at the ends for handles—to whatever you're using to keep the tires together. For additional resistance, either add more tires or insert tied-down dumbbells inside the bottom tire.

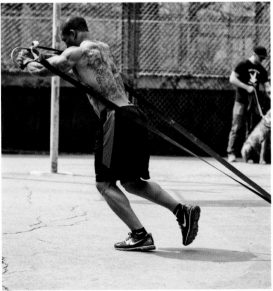

TIRE PRESS
Holding the handles in a neutral grip in bench press position at chest level, walk forward until you feel tension in the straps. Press the straps forward to lockout, then step forward and repeat.

Chapter 10

ATTACK YOUR WEAK POINTS, HEAD TO TOE, WITH THIS PHYSIQUE TROUBLESHOOTING GUIDE.

SPOT ON TRAINING

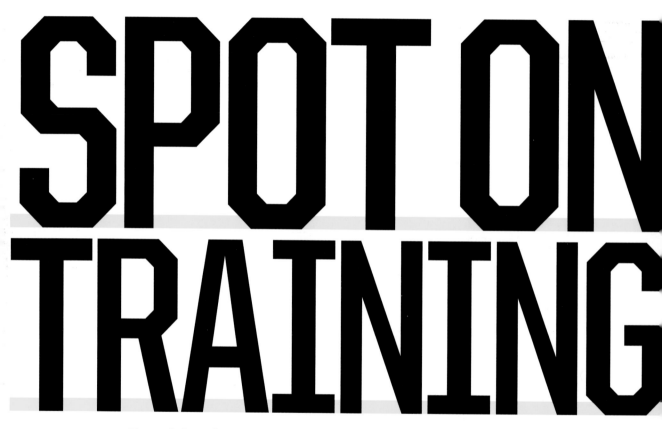

Let's face facts: You've got weaknesses. We all do. We're human. And when it comes to our physiques, nitpicking those weaknesses comes with the territory: Pecs not quite as separated as you'd like. Triceps looking more like half a horseshoe than the whole thing. Quads not displaying that telltale teardrop.

To turn such weaknesses into strengths, we've compiled a list of seven of the most troublesome areas for guys, and the best exercises for bringing them up to par—and beyond. Attack these weak points with abandon and you'll have a spot-on physique in no time.

INCLINE CABLE FLYE
Connect two D-handles to the low pulleys of a cable-crossover station. Set an adjustable bench to a 45-degree angle (or lower) and position it between the cables so that they're in line with your chest. Lie on the bench and begin by holding the handles with your arms out at your sides (elbows slightly bent) and your palms facing up. Contract your pecs to pull your arms up and together over your chest until your hands meet, maintaining the slight bend in your elbows throughout. Slowly return to the start position by lowering your arms back out to your sides until your wrists come to about shoulder level or slightly above.

BEHIND-THE-BACK CABLE C
Face away from a low-pulley cable station
your right heel aligned with the pulley. With
right hand, grasp a D-handle and allow you
to extend behind you at about a 30-degree
from your torso. Keeping your upper arm f
curl the handle and squeeze at the

WEAK SPOT No.1:

BICEPS PEAK

There's not a guy alive who doesn't want a more impressive biceps peak. And while the amount of peak you have on your biceps is to some degree genetically predetermined, that doesn't mean you can't drastically improve what you've got. The key is exercise selection. The majority of the peak that pops up when you flex your biceps is the long (outer) head. You can better isolate it by performing curls with arms behind the body, as in behind-the-back cable curls or incline dumbbell curls. Another useful technique is to curl with the arms turned toward the body, as with concentration curls and close-grip barbell curls.

BICEPS PEAK WORKOUT

EXERCISE	SETS	REPS	RES
Barbell Curl*	3	6-8	1-2 m
Behind-the-back Cable Curl	3	10-12	1-2 m
Preacher Curl	3	10-12	1-2 m
Dumbbell Concentration Curl	3	12-15	**

*Do the first two sets with a narrow grip (less t
shoulder width) to emphasize the biceps long
head.

**Don't take an official rest—go back and forth
from arm to arm until three sets per arm have
been completed.

WEAK SPOT No.2:

UPPER INNER PECS

Your chest is usually hidden. But a V-neck shirt or tank top shows off one area—the upper section of the inner pecs. If they're flat, your physique loses something. This is a hard-to-reach spot for many guys to develop, and if you're focusing on it with incline dumbbell flyes, you're missing out. Switching to cables provides the continuous tension you need when the hands touch at the top. For incline presses, use dumbbells—the arc they allow you to form as you press up and together better targets the upper, inner pecs than a barbell does.

UPPER INNER PECS WORKOUT

EXERCISE	SETS	REPS	RES
Incline Dumbbell Press	3-4	6-8	1-2 m
Barbell Bench Press	3-4	6-8	1-2 m
Incline Cable Flye	3-4	10-12	1 mi
Cable Crossover	3-4	12-15	1 mi

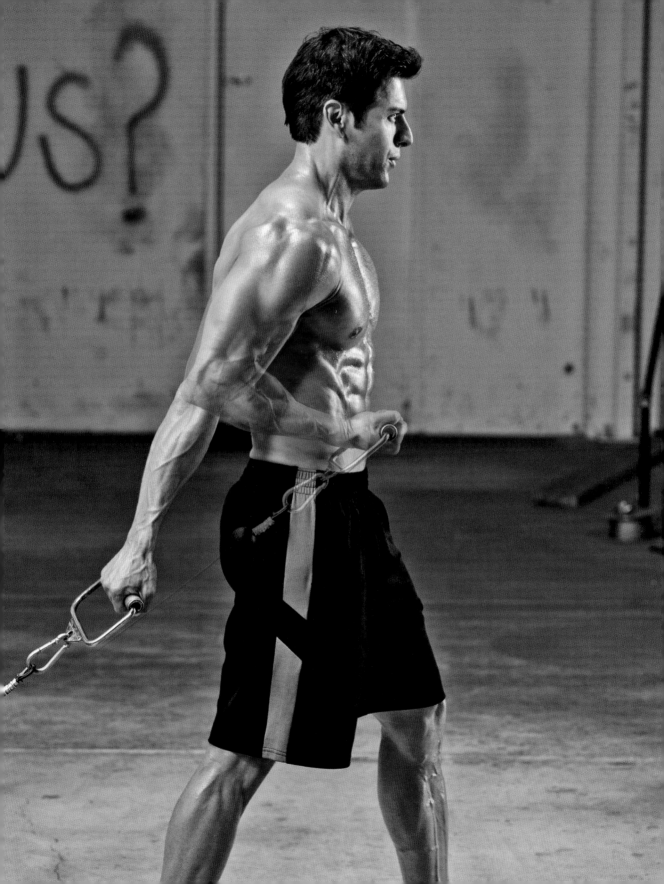

DUMBBELL TRICEPS KICKBACK
Press your right arm tight against your side, with the upper arm parallel to the floor and your forearm hanging straight down. Keeping your upper arm stationary, contract your triceps to extend your elbow. Flex the triceps hard for a second, then return to start position.

WEAK SPOT No. 3:
TRICEPS LATERAL HEAD

The triceps lateral head makes up the part of the horseshoe that runs down the side of the arm. When it has a lot of mass it adds width to the arms, and when it's well defined it makes the triceps look as if they're carved out of stone. Although doing pressdowns with a rope is a serviceable enough way to hit the lateral head, a recent study commissioned by the American Council on Exercise (ACE) by the University of Wisconsin-La Crosse showed that, for this purpose, dumbbell kickbacks blow rope and straight-bar pressdowns away.

TRICEPS LATERAL HEAD WORKOUT

EXERCISE	SETS	REPS	REST
Close-grip Bench Press	3	6-8	1-2 mi
Dumbbell Triceps Kickback	3	10-12	1-2 mi
Dumbbell Overhead Triceps Extension	3	10-12	1-2 mi
One-arm Reverse-grip Triceps Pressdown	3	12-15	-

QUADRICEPS "TEARDROP"

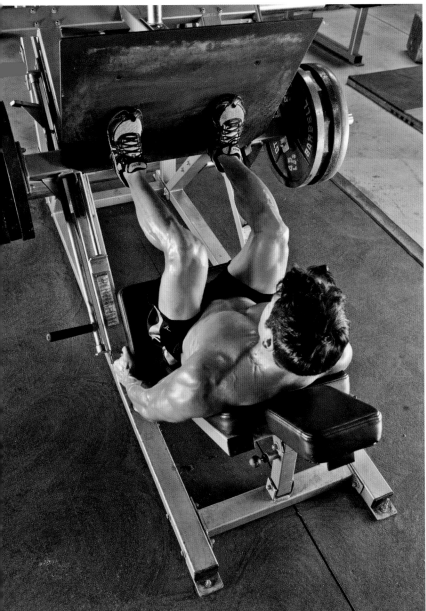

Training legs is important for overall strength and muscle mass—and for not being that guy whose upper arms are bigger than his thighs. But short-shorts went out of style in the '80s. What's fashionable today are long-inseam shorts that cover up the quads almost completely. One area that often remains visible, however, is the vastus medialis (teardrop) muscle that extends down the inner side of the knee. There are a few exercises and techniques you can do to place more focus on this area. First, don't go so heavy on barbell squats: One study found that keeping weight lighter and reps relatively high during squats put the most focus on the quads and less on the hamstrings. Exercises that specifically target the teardrop are leg presses (shown in another study to emphasize the vastus medialis the most of all leg movements) and leg extensions in which the feet are turned outward.

"TEARDROP" WORKOUT

EXERCISE	SETS	REPS	REST
Squat	4	10-15	1-2 min.
Leg Press	4	8-10	1-2 min.
Leg Extension*	4	12-15	1-2 min.

*Do the first two sets with your feet rotated out, to emphasize the teardrop muscle.

SEATED LEG CURL
Sit in a seated leg curl machine with your knees just past the bench. Contract your hamstrings to curl your lower legs under you, bringing your feet as close to the bottom of the bench as possible. Hold for a second and squeeze your hamstrings hard; return to the start position.

WEAK SPOT No. 5:
REAR DELTS/MIDDLE TRAPS

Possessing a thick upper back and rear delts is a great way to fill out a T-shirt. Unfortunately, it's more common to see a guy with big pecs and front deltoids but flat muscles on the opposite side. Don't be that guy. The upper back is composed mainly of the middle traps, which work together with the rear delts during exercises that bring the arms from front to back, pulling perpendicular to the body. The face pull is such a move, and one that will provide great balance to the incline presses and flyes you do on chest day. In the workout below, you'll do the face pull after all other deltoid exercises, as it's a great segue between delt and upper-traps training.

REAR DELTS/MIDDLE TRAPS WORKOUT

EXERCISE	SETS	REPS	REST
Barbell Shoulder Press	3-4	6-8	1-2 m
Dumbbell Lateral Raise	3-4	10-12	1-2 m
Dumbbell Front Raise	3-4	10-12	1-2 m
Face Pull	3-4	8-10	1-2 m
Barbell Shrug	3-4	6-8	1-2 m

WEAK SPOT No. 6:
INNER HAMSTRINGS

It's a common misconception that there's only one muscle on the back of thighs. But while the biceps femoris makes up the majority of your hamstring mass, there are actually three different muscles comprising the hammies—the other two are the semitendinosus and semimembranosus, which make up the inner hamstrings. If you do only lying leg curls, your outer hamstrings likely overshadow your inners. The below workout, which you can perform immediately after the quad routine for Weak Spot No. 6, will help fix this imbalance. Romanian deadlifts build overall mass, while research shows that seated leg curls place more emphasis on the inner hams. When doing lying leg curls, turn your feet in further.

INNER HAMSTRINGS WORKOUT

EXERCISE	SETS	REPS	REST
Romanian Deadlift	3-4	8-10	1-2 min.
Seated Leg Curl	3	8-10	1-2 min.
Lying Leg Curl (feet turned in)	3	8-10	1-2 min.

WEAK SPOT No. 7:
LOWER LATS

Having massive lats makes you look impressive from behind. What looks less than impressive, however, are lats that are all up top with little to nothing down low—we call this "high-lats syndrome."

Impressive lats need to be wide and thick from your armpits to your waist. Exercises that bring your elbows from out at your sides to down toward your waist, such as wide-grip lat pulldowns, work the upper lats well.

Focusing on lo lats requires movements th bring your elbo from in front o your body dow like straight-ar and reverse-gr pulldowns.

LOWER LATS WORKOUT

EXERCISE	SETS	REPS	REST
Straight-arm Pulldown	3-4	12-15	1-2 min.
Reverse-grip Pulldown	3-4	8-10	1-2 min.
Wide-grip Pulldown	3-4	10-12	1-2 min.
Barbell Bentover Row	3-4	8-10	1-2 min.

STRAIGHT-ARM PULLDOWN
Stand behind a lat-pulldown machine with your knees slightly bent. G the bar with an overhand grip and your arms shoulder-width apart. In position, your arms should be straight out in front of you with your ha above shoulder height. From here, use your lats to pull your arms dow and bring the bar to your upper thighs.

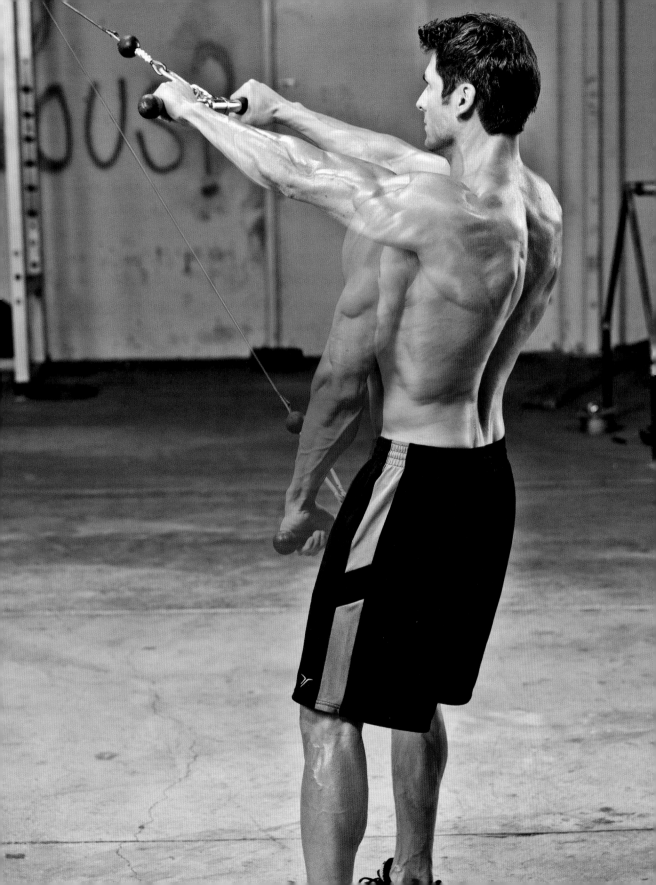

Chapter 11

THESE MUSCLE-BUILDING MOVES HAVE BEEN ABSENT FROM YOUR WORKOUTS FOR TOO LONG—MAYBE FOREVER. IT'S TIME FOR A PROPER INTRODUCTION.

THE NINE BEST EXERCISES YOU'RE NOT DOING

Sometimes the best exercise is the one you're not doing. And why, exactly, is such a great move not part of your training? Probably one of two reasons: a) you don't know it exists, or b) it's so challenging that you'd rather skip it and do something easier. The following nine exercises are ones we feel every physique-conscious guy should practice. Some you've heard of but are ignoring, and others are so unique we bet they've never crossed your mind. Either way, it's time to add these moves to your repertoire.

FRONT SQUAT

CONTRIBUTOR: Phil Heath, reigning Mr. Olympia

WHY YOU SHOULD BE DOING IT: "Front squats have really helped quad development, especially when I was preparing for the Sandman," says Heath. "Most people don't do front squats, because they're uncomfortable and there are easier alternatives, but to really add size to the quads, they're a must."

HOW TO DO IT: In a power rack, place the bar across your front deltoids with your forearms crossed in front of you and hands gripping the bar. Unrack the bar, step back, and begin the set standing straight up with your feet about shoulder-width apart and your elbows pointed straight ahead, not downward. Keeping a slight arch in your lower back, squat down over your heels, keeping your elbows up until your thighs reach parallel with the floor. Press up through your heels until your knees are extended but not locked out.

2 ARCHED-BACK PULLUP

CONTRIBUTOR:

Martin Rooney, CEO of trainingforwarriors.com and author of *Warrior Cardio: The Revolutionary Metabolic Training System for Burning Fat, Building Muscle, and Getting Fit*

WHY YOU SHOULD BE DOING IT:

"This exercise involves both a vertical and horizontal pull from the upper body—most pulling moves involve only one or the other," Rooney says. "It maximizes core and abdominal recruitment. So, the arched-back pullup hits about as much total muscle as any lift."

HOW TO DO IT:

Drape a neutral-grip cable rowing handle over a pullup bar. Grasp the handle with both hands and start from a hanging position, arms fully extended. Pull your chest toward the hand while also lifting your hips up and letting your head travel back so that at the top of the rep, your chest touches your hands and your torso is roughly parallel with the floor.

3. CRUSH-GRIP DUMBBELL BENCH PRESS

CONTRIBUTOR: Jim Smith, C.S.C.S., owner of Diesel Strength & Conditioning (*dieselsc.com*), member of the *Livestrong.com* advisory board

WHY YOU SHOULD BE DOING IT: "'Crushing' the dumbbells together while slowing the tempo increases the tension across the chest, shoulders, triceps, and upper back," says Jim Smith, C.S.C.S. "More time under tension will immediately increase the muscle-building and natural hormone-release effect."

HOW TO DO IT: Sit on the end of a flat bench holding a pair of dumbbells. Lie back and hold the dumbbells over your chest, arms extended, with the insides of the dumbbells touching. As you lower the weights toward your chest, press them together as hard as possible. When they reach your chest, lift the weights back up, still pressing them together. Keep the rep speed slow.

4. WIDE-GRIP UPRIGHT ROW

CONTRIBUTOR: Justin Grinnell, C.S.C.S., co-owner of State of Fitness in East Lansing, MI (*mystateoffitness.com*)

WHY YOU SHOULD BE DOING IT: Wide-grip upright rows can be a great deltoid builder if used correctly, Justin Grinnell says. "Doin them with the wider grip will take the traps out of the movement," he says, "and you'll hit the delts better than you would if you were using a narrow grip." But if you have shoulder impingement issues proceed with caution.

HOW TO DO IT: Stand holding a barbell in front of your thighs wit your arms fully extended and your hands outside shoulder width. With your knees slightly bent, pull the bar straight up your body, bending your elbows, until it reaches chest height. As you lift the bar, don't let your shoulders shrug up; keep them depressed to maintain tension in the delts. Hold the contraction at the top for a count, then lower back down.

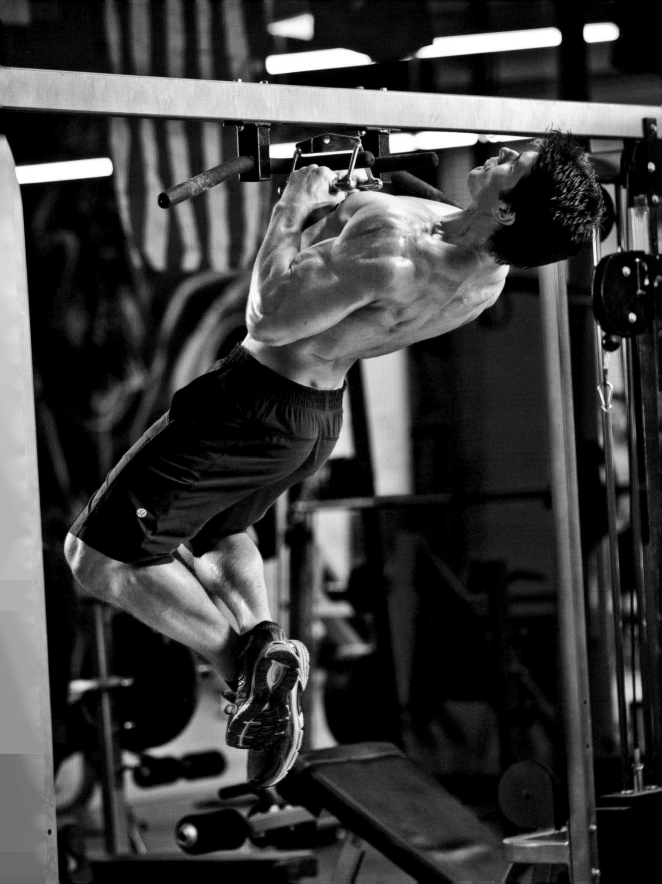

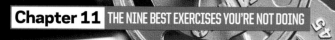

OVERHEAD SQUAT

CONTRIBUTOR:
Brian Strump, D.C., owner
of CrossFit Steele Creek
and Premier Health & Rehab
Solutions in Charlotte, NC
(crossfitsteelecreek.com)

WHY YOU SHOULD BE DOING IT:

"The overhead squat is not an exercise you should be skipping," Strump says. "It integrates functional strength, flexibility, and core and shoulder stability. With so much going on, the overhead squat elicits a hormonal response that builds muscle and burns fat."

HOW TO DO IT:

Grasp a relatively light Olympic barbell in a power rack with a very wide, overhand grip (aka snatch grip), with your feet shoulder-width apart, your back flat, and your chest out. Push-press the bar overhead so you're in standing position, arms fully extended, shoulder blades squeezed together. The bar should be slightly behind your head, not directly over or in front of it. Maintaining this bar position, slowly squat down as if sitting on a stool, keeping your chest out, until your thighs reach parallel with the floor. Press through your heels to stand back up to the start position.

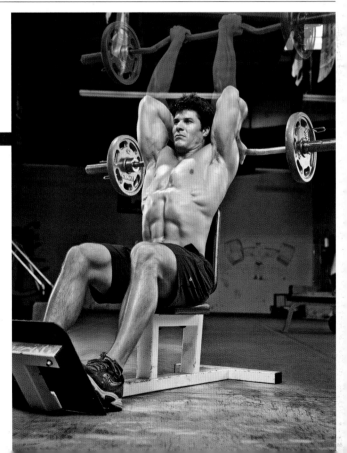

6. SEATED REVERSE-GRIP OVERHEAD TRICEPS EXTENSION

CONTRIBUTOR: Ray Wetterlund III, C.S.C.S., USA weightlifting coach and celebrity personal trainer in La Jolla, CA (rw3fitness.com)

WHY YOU SHOULD BE DOING IT: "The long head of the triceps tends to get neglected," Wetterlund says, "primarily because it responds best to heavy loads and overhead movements, which people often leave out of their arm routines. This is why the seated overhead extension is my go-to move for bringing up the long head."

HOW TO DO IT: Sit on a low-back seat or bench and hold an EZ-curl bar overhead with your arms extended and an underhand grip (palms and forearms facing behind you) inside shoulder width. Keeping your upper arms stationary and your elbows in tight, bend your elbows to slowly lower the bar until your elbows reach 90 degrees of flexion. Contract your triceps to extend your elbows to full lockout at the top.

7. BICEPS LADDER

CONTRIBUTOR: Jim Stoppani, Ph.D., former *M&F* senior science editor and host of the popular video series *M&F Raw!* at *muscle-andfitness.com*

WHY YOU SHOULD BE DOING IT: On top of the crazy pump you'll get, the ladder has a host of other benefits."The biceps ladder is a great mass builder," says Jim Stoppani. "First, it allows you to go heavier than you could with standard curls (using your own body weight). Second, you're focusing on the negative of each rep, which will further stimulate growth. And finally, the 'ladder' aspect of the lift functions like a dropset, increasing your total number of reps to maximize blood flow to the biceps. One trip up the ladder and your biceps will be screaming."

HOW TO DO IT: Set a bar in a power rack just above arm's length from the floor. Grab the bar with a shoulder-width, underhand grip with your body hanging underneath it just above the floor, in a straight line from head to toe. Starting with your arms fully extended, curl yourself up as high as possible, bringing your forehead to the bar. Do as many reps as you can, then raise the bar one setting and repeat. Keep raising the bar until you can't perform any more reps.

8. SEATED ROTATION

CONTRIBUTOR: Gunnar Peterson, C.S.C.S., trainer to celebs su as Sylvester Stallone, Bruce Willis, and Tom Brady

WHY YOU SHOULD BE DOING IT: "Life and sport happen in the transverse plane, like when you put on your seatbelt or swing a b says celebrity trainer Gunnar Peterson. "You need to train that wa in the gym. Like the commercial says, 'Keep crunching,' but add ir some side-to-side rotation to do everything better."

HOW TO DO IT: Sit on the floor holding a weight or medicine ball with both hands in front of you, elbows slightly bent. Start with y knees bent 90 degrees and feet on the floor (advanced trainees can raise their feet off the floor). Rotate the weight from one hip the other in a continuous side-to-side motion, following the weigh with your eyes and allowing your shoulders to rotate. Try to keep your legs from swaying side to side during the movement. It's not just difficult in terms of coordination; it will also give your stabiliz muscles a ton of extra work.

9 GOOD MORNING

CONTRIBUTOR:

Guillermo Escalante, C.S.C.S., bodybuilder and co-owner of SportsPros Personal Training/Physical Therapy Center in Claremont, CA (*4sportspros.com*)

WHY YOU SHOULD BE DOING IT:

"Good mornings are a really effective exercise that most people don't do," Escalante says. "They target the larger posterior chain muscles (glutes, hamstrings, and para-spinals), which can help you improve your strength in lifts like the deadlift and squat, as well as decrease your risk of lower-back injury."

HOW TO DO IT:

Stand with feet hip- to shoulder-width apart, holding a relatively light barbell acros your upper traps. Keeping your back flat and knees slightly bent , slowly bend your hips back to lower your torso toward the floor. Whe your torso reaches parallel with the floor, reverse the motion to return to the standing position.

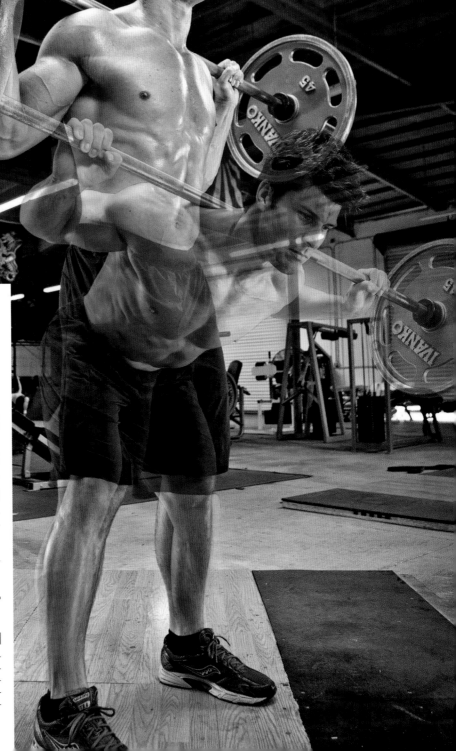

JST DO IT

nt to get after these nine
eat exercises ASAP? Try this
per-body/lower-body two-day
it for a workout your muscles
ll never see coming.

AY 1
PER BODY

KERCISE	SETS	REPS
ush-grip Dumbbell nch Press	3-4	8-10
PERSET WITH		
rbell Bentover Row	3-4	8-10
ched-back Pullup	3	6
PERSET WITH		
cline Barbell Press	3	6
de-grip Upright Row	3-4	10-12
ated Reverse-grip erhead Triceps tension	4	10-12
ceps Ladder	1	Up the ladder to failure

AY 2
WER BODY + CORE

KERCISE	SETS	REPS
ont Squat	4	6-8
erhead Squat	3	8-10
od Morning	3	10-12
ing or Seated Leg Curl	3	12
ated Rotation	3-4	15-20
nging Leg Raise	3-4	12

SHOW-OFF MUSCLE

Flip through the pages of this book and you'll come across dozens of shredded guys in various stages of undress. They're typically shirtless, wearing workout trunks or compression shorts. While this is effective in showing what *M&F* can do for your physique, it's probably not how you plan to dress during summer. When you're scoping out the local talent while sipping zero-carb mojitos at the bar, letting it all hang out isn't really an option unless you're a world-class narcissist. And although we're sure there are a few of you out there, the rest of us will spend our summers wearing the uniform: T-shirts, cargo shorts, and flip-flops.

People can see a great physique no matter what you wear, but with typical summer guy attire, the only muscles you're directly showing the world are your forearms, calves, and neck. On the following pages, you'll find the formula for putting the finishing touches on everything you've worked for during the winter: forearms that pop from the mere thought of twisting a bottle cap, a neck that stretches the rings of your T-shirts, and calves that could be mistaken for cows.

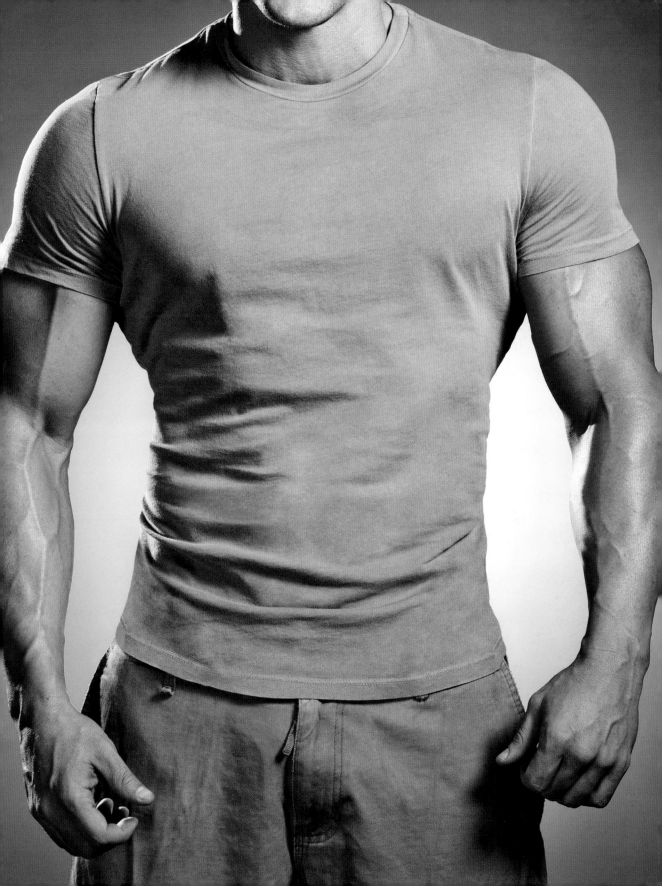

IT'S NOT JUST FOR LOOKS

In the gym, you're only as strong as your weakest link, so you can't expect massive leg development or a huge squat without a solid set of calves. Likewise, you're going to have a tough time developing solid pecs if you have weak hands and skinny forearms. And that barn-door shoulder width and V-taper we're all after can't possibly be attained with a pencil-thin neck as your foundation. These muscles need work, especially if you haven't been hitting them directly, and the benefits of training the "ancillary" muscle groups are myriad. In fact, your body wants to maintain some level of equilibrium when it comes to size, so if you focus on these forgotten groups, your toil will result in quick gains in both strength and mass.

These muscles are relatively small, so in terms of weight-room performance, they're just links in a much longer chain. What you want, however, is for your neck, forearms, and calves to be up for Best Supporting Actor nominations—as opposed to playing forgettable bit parts that contribute little to your plot. It's neither efficient nor effective to schedule a dedicated day for these character actors, though, so the idea is to elicit as much growth as possible from your main movements—followed by accessory exercises designed to maintain that momentum.

HOW IT WORKS

Focusing on these areas will take some additional work, which means you'll need time for extra exercises and longer workouts on certain days. For example, on one of your lower-body days, you'll squat, then train your calves, and then train everything else. On back day, you'll perform deadlifts with Grip4orce (rubber sleeves you'll slide on the bar; grip4orce.com), followed by the rest of your forearm workout, then transition into whatever else you have planned for that day. Plan ahead, schedule your time accordingly, and use this template for the next eight weeks.

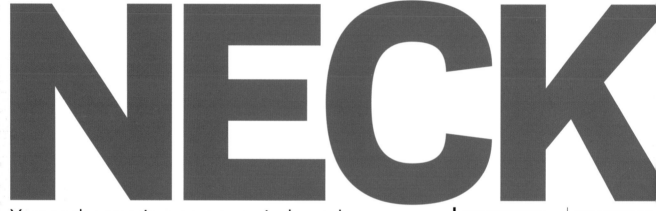

NECK

Your neck comprises seven cervical vertebrae—the top part of the bony column that leads down to your spine. Your cervical vertebrae are the smallest units in the column (think of each separate vertebra as being approximately the size of an Oreo Double Stuf cookie). They're also among the most important, since each individual vertebra has considerable influence on a different basic human function—including sight, facial movement, and the use of your hands. Your cervical vertebrae are worth protecting and developing for reasons far more profound than a desire to stop popping your collar to hide your scrawny stack of dimes.

Because your cervical vertebrae are relatively fragile, the key to effective neck training is adherence to the less-is-more philosophy. You'll incorporate your neck training into a lower-body or shoulder day once per week, avoiding working yourself to a point where you can't look from side to side without turning your entire body.

CHIN-BACK GOOD MORNING

With a barbell on your shoulders, pull your chin back as far as you can to put your neck in a tight, anatomically correct cervical position. With your knees slightly bent and your lower back firm and straight, bend at the waist until your upper body is nearly parallel to the floor, then use your lower back and hamstrings to return to the start position.

OVERHEAD SHRUG

Grasp the bar with your hands shoulder-width apart, or slightly wider, and press it overhead. With your arms fully extended and your elbows locked out, shrug the bar up and down for reps.

FOUR-WAY NECK MACHINE

If your gym has one of these, you're fortunate. These units differ in terms of how your body is positioned, but make sure to work your neck from all four angles for an equal number of sets and reps. Don't have access to this machine? Use a neck harness or simply do isometric holds by pressing your head against your hand.

FAT-GRIP SHRUG
Stand with your feet shoulder-width apart. Hold the grips with your hands just outside your thighs and shrug your shoulders as high as you can. Hold for a second at the top, then return to the starting position and repeat. Using Grip4orce or a similar grip sleeve on the bar will give this exercise the dual benefit of hitting the forearms as well as the neck.

CK (SHOULDER DAY)

ERCISE	SETS	REPS	REST
d Morning	3-5	5	90 sec.
rhead Shrug	3	15	60 sec.
grip Shrug	5	25	60 sec.
-way			
k Machine*	3	20	60 sec.

*stitute neck harness or isometric work;
0 reps in each direction.*

FOREAI

Your forearms let the world know you've put some serious time into developing your physique. A well-developed, vein-laden set of forearms demonstrates that you've either been lifting weights seriously or engaging in heavy manual labor on a regular basis for a long time. Either way, the rest of the room will know you're not someone to mess with.

There are myriad options for bringing your forearms up to speed. In this program, we're advocating a significant amount of grip work through the use of Grip4orce grips. If you can't get a set of these, use towels to simulate fat grips where your hands hold the barbell. For now, think of huge forearms and a crushing grip as partners. You can't have one without the other.

GRIP4ORCE DOUBLE OVERHA DEADLIFT

With a loaded barb on the floor, bend down and grasp th bar overhand-style with the grips plac just outside your fe Bend your knees, c your butt, and kee the bar as close to your body as possi raise it in a straigh line until you're sta ing upright. Use th touch-and-go met between reps (dor rest the bar on the floor) to increase y time under tension

GRIP4ORCE REVERSE-GRIP C

Place the grips on a loaded barbell and them with an overh grip, letting the bar straight down at yo waist. Curl the bar i an arc as far as you toward your face, h at the top for a sec then slowly return start position.

FAT-GRIP INVERTED ROW

Lay a barbell acros the spotter bars o power rack or squa rack. Lie on your b with your feet elev and hold the barbe with the grips, wit your hands should width apart. Keepi your body in a stra rigid line, pull your up until your chest touches the bar, h for a second, then return to a dead hang position.

FOREARMS (BACK DAY)

EXERCISE	SETS	REPS	REST
Double-overhand Deadlift	3-5	5	90 sec.
Reverse-grip Curl	3	25	60 sec.
Plate Pinch	3	ALAP*	60 sec.
Fat-grip Inverted Row	3	AMAP**	60 sec.

*As long as possible
**As many as possible

RMS

STANDING CALF RAISE

Stand on the balls of your feet in a calf press machine with the pads on your shoulders. Using your calves and ankles, raise yourself as high as you can, hold for a second, then return to the start position.

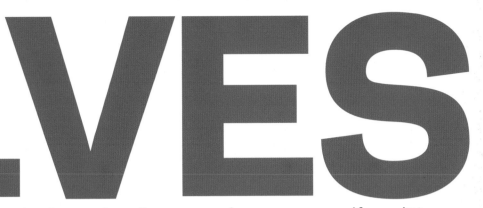

ALVES

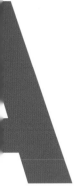

K SQUAT
a barbell across
shoulders, stand
your feet shoul-
width apart. Keep-
our upper body
, your lower back
, and your head up,
 your descent by
ing your hips back
downward. To fully
ge your calves,
rm a full Olympic
t—going well
 parallel.

KING
OE LUNGE
ing a pair of
bbells at your
s, take a long step
ard, landing on the
of your foot and
ing your heel up.
 your front knee
descend until your
 knee touches
ground, then push
 up and repeat
 your other leg.

AIGHT-LEG
P ROPE
 rope, but restrict
pend in your knees
bounce off the
 of your feet, using
your ankles and
es to move your
 up and down.

For both aesthetics and performance, there are two calf conditions you want to avoid like the plague: nankles and cankles. With nankles, you've got nothing. Your ankles and calves are simply one big bone attachment with no muscle anywhere. Cankles are even worse. This means your lower leg is just a giant, undefined tube of uniform circumference from your knees to your ankles. There's no separation, and the only immediate solution is to throw on a baggy pair of pants. Quickly.

Take a look at the calves of any professional athlete—especially those of football players, sprinters, and boxers. Their calves ooze potential energy, literally blooming from the popliteal fossa (the back of the knee) down with every step, even when they're just walking casually. This is what you want: for your calves to announce your athleticism. At any given moment they'll say, you can run fast, jump high, and calf press tractor trailers.

LVES (LEG DAY)

ERCISE	SETS	REPS	REST
k Squat	5	8	120 sec.
king toe Lunge	3	8 (each)	90 sec.
nding f Raise	3	15	60 sec.
aight-leg p Rope	5	60 sec.	60 sec.

THE METABOLIC WORKOUT

The excess fat on your body is a lot like a nut attached to a rusted-out bolt. You want to twist it off. You need to twist it off. Chances are, you've tried everything you can think of to unscrew it, but nothing ever seems to work. It's stuck—and so are you.

When this happens, any machine or auto repair shop worth its salt has just the last-resort solution on hand to get things moving: a blowtorch. When you blowtorch a rusted nut-and-bolt arrangement, the intense heat breaks the bond created by the rust, and it melts things down to a point where the nut can easily be removed.

That's how it works with fat loss, too. When all else fails—when your diet and cardio "solutions" aren't solving a blessed thing—it's time to break out your own blowtorch and get the lard off once and for all. We're about to show you how to do this with a healthy dose of intensity by adding metabolic circuit training to your regimen.

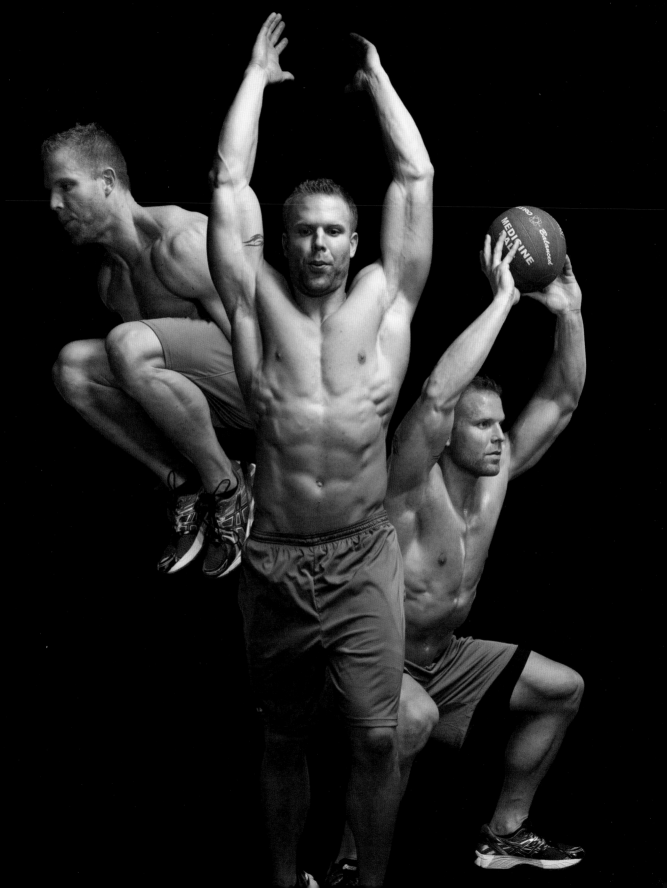

EPOC EPIC

You may have heard about excess post-exercise oxygen consumption in the past. EPOC is the gas tank that powers your fat-stripping blowtorch, because when the type of training we're advocating here induces an "oxygen debt," it can increase your metabolic rate for up to 16 hours after you train. This means that when you're done working out—while you're at school, at work, or sleeping—your body is still looking to consume fuel sources for the oxygen it needs to restore itself to a resting state of equilibrium. The good news for you is that it does this primarily through raiding fat stores.

"The EPOC effect does what steady-state cardio can't do," says Ryan Whitton, a strength coach in Austin, TX. "You still need some steady-state in your program to enhance recovery and strengthen your heart, but when it comes to stripping fat off your body, nothing works like circuit training to manipulate the speed at which your metabolism burns."

Research has shown that the EPOC effect increases along with the intensity level of the type of exercise you're performing. So, while you may burn more calories during a low-impact 45-minute treadmill session, you'll affect your metabolic rate in a far more profound way if you throw in two or three short-yet-intense 10-minute metabolic circuits per week.

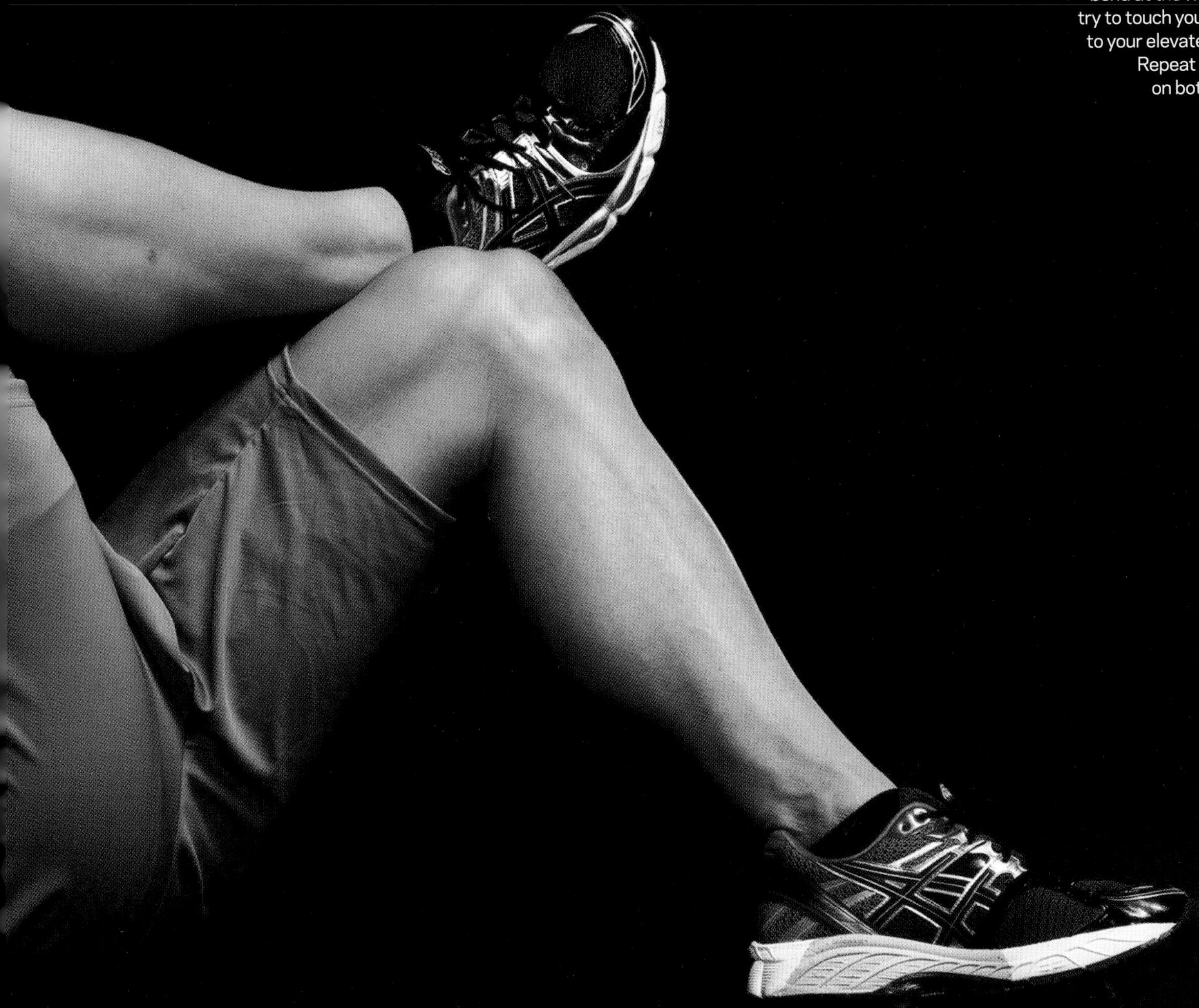

FIGURE-4 SITUP
Lie on the floor on your back, with your knees bent. Cross one leg over the other so the outside of your elevated leg, just above your ankle, is resting on your other leg just above the knee. Place your hand opposite your elevated leg behind your head, then bend at the waist and try to touch your elbow to your elevated knee. Repeat for reps on both sides.

TUCK JUMP

Stand with your feet shoulder-width apart, with your knees bent and your hands and elbows in an athletic position. Jump as high as you can, tuck your knees into your chest, then land as softly as possible. Gather yourself and repeat for reps.

SIMPLY SHREDDED

Whether you're willing to admit it or not, metabolic-style training is fun despite its high degree of difficulty. The workouts move quickly, the exercises are constantly changing, and it forces you to use your entire body as a unit—the way it's intended to move—instead of performing the same repetitive moves for set periods of time, à la steady-state cardio.

You can also train this way anywhere. Whether you're traveling, pressed for time, or you'd rather wait until you're home from the gym to receive your metabolic ass kicking, most of the exercises in this set of workouts involve just your body weight—with the rest utilizing dumbbells, the weight of which can remain constant. In other words, you won't need a ton of time, space, or gear—just the desire to shred those last bits of winter body fat and a plan to complete the job.

"If I showed you someone who trained with these circuits for an extended period of time," says Whitton, an experienced amateur fighter who favors MMA-style training for his clients, "you'd see how they look and perform and you'd want those types of results for yourself."

From a standing position, move forward by driving your right knee into your chest to begin the skip. Land on the ball of your left foot, then immediately descend into a lunge with your right foot forward. From this position, explode into another skip, this time leading with your left knee. Repeat for 20 yards down and back.

WORKOUTS

Two or three times per week, choose one of the following workouts and perform as many rounds as you can.

WORKOUT 1

EXERCISE	REPS
Medicine Ball Overhead Squat	10
Tuck Jump	10
Scissor Lunge	10
Skip and Scoop	20 yards there and back

WORKOUT 2

EXERCISE	REPS
Burpee with Tuck Jump	10
Pushup	10
Mountain Climber	10
Figure-4 Situp	10 each side

WORKOUT 3

EXERCISE	REPS
DB Burpee Clean and Press	10
DB Thruster	10
DB Snatch	10 each hand
DB Woodchopper	10 each side

MOUNTAIN CLIMBER

Stay in a pushup position and forcefully kick your left knee to your chest, landing the ball of your left foot on the ground. Then, bring your right knee to your chest and return your right foot to the start position. Repeat as though you're running in place.

HOW IT WORKS

Perform circuits consecutively with no breaks between exercises; then rest for 60 to 90 seconds between rounds—crank out as many rounds as you can. This doesn't mean you should be hitting these circuits every day, however. For most people, two or three hard metabolic circuits per week will suffice, because you can't recover from this level of intensity in just 24 hours. Additionally, the hampered recovery levels caused by overtraining with metabolic circuits will negatively affect your strength and mass-building workouts, because you won't be recovered enough to make significant progress if you're consistently running yourself into the ground with anaerobic torture. Your body can't hold up to it, and your returns will begin to diminish in short order.

"The best way to get this done is to leave at least 48 to 72 hours between workouts," says Whitton. "Too many guys think that if they're not in a constant state of exhaustion, that they're not going to burn enough fat, but this isn't the case. These workouts are about quality as much as quantity. I'd rather see my clients work themselves to exhaustion twice per week and take the rest the days off than train like this every day, because all the positive changes to your body happen during recovery periods."

Now, this won't be an easy six weeks. You'll essentially be working yourself to the bone twice per week—getting more rounds in each time out—in order to accelerate your results, so this isn't a "less is more" training scenario. That's a good thing according to Whitton. "Along with basking in the glow of the EPOC effect," he says, "when you eventually get off the floor and leave the gym, you know you put in a hard day's work, and that's worth all the effort."

DUMBBELL SNATCH

Stand with your feet shoulder-width apart and your knees slightly bent, holding a dumbbell in front of your thighs in each hand. Extend your ankles, knees, and hips to explosively raise both dumbbells overhead. You should feel like you're trying to throw them through the ceiling.

DUMBBELL BURPEE CLEAN AND PRESS

Holding a pair of dumbbells, perform a burpee except without the tuck jump. Once you've returned to the start position, explosively clean the dumbbells to shoulder level, then press them over your head. Lower the weights to your sides and repeat.

MEDICINE BALL OVERHEAD SQUAT

Hold a medicine ball with both hands extended directly over your head. Push your hips backward and descend into a below-parallel squat, keeping your core tight and the medicine ball high. Explosively return to the start position and repeat.

SCISSOR JUMP

From a standing position, jump into a forward lunge, with your left leg forward, your right leg back, and your arms bent in a sprinter's position. From the bottom of the movement, jump up, and in one motion, land with your right leg forward and your left leg back.

DUMBBELL THRUSTER

From a standing position, hold two dumbbells at shoulder level as though you're about to press them overhead. Push your hips back and descend into a squat. From the bottom position, use your upward momentum to drive the dumbbells explosively over your head. Lower them to the start position and repeat.

BURPEE WITH TUCK JUMP

From a standing position, squat down, place your hands on the floor and kick your feet back together so you're in a pushup position. Rapidly bring your feet back to the squat position, then explode upward into a tuck jump, bringing your knees into your chest. Repeat.

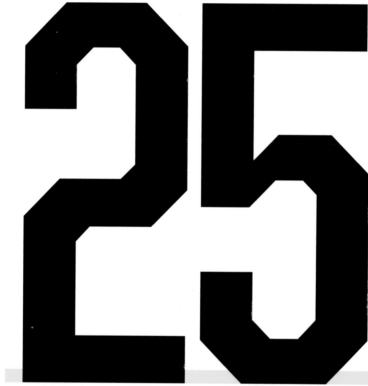

25
TIPS FOR MORE MUSCLE AND SUPER STRENGTH

There's nothing wrong with following any of the programs in this book exactly as written. You'll get great results doing so. But sometimes it helps to have an extra trick up your sleeve to gain an edge in the gym and bust through a plateau. And that's what you have in this chapter: 25 tips that most hardcore lifters are familiar with and the average Joe isn't. Use a few (or all) of these from time to time in your training and you'll have an added advantage over that everyday Joe.

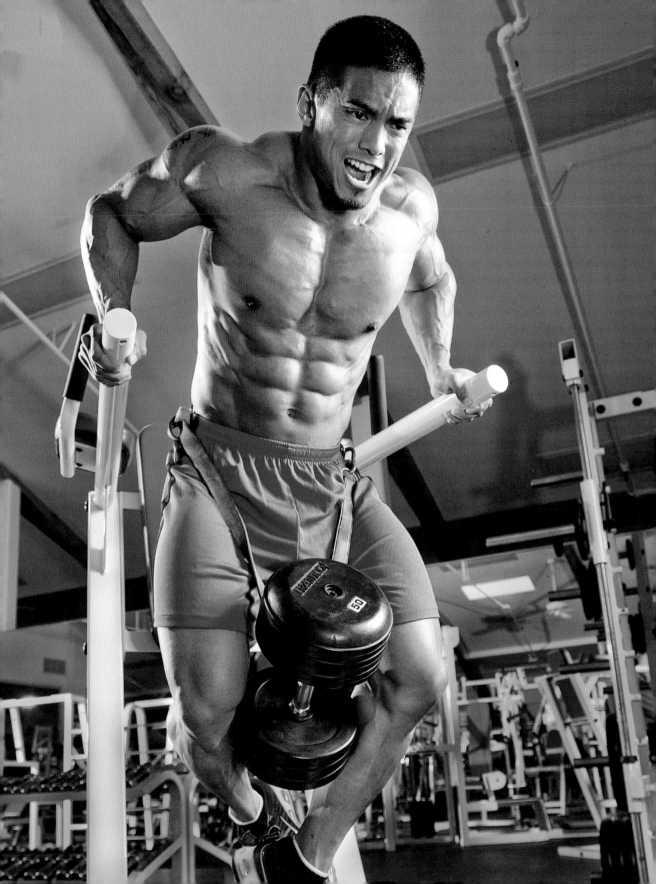

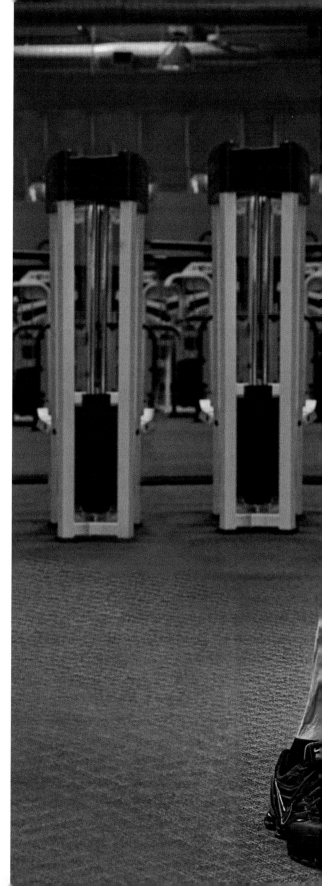

1.
LOSE THE SHOES

Lift barefoot, if possible, or in minimalist footwear like Vibram Five-Fingers shoes, wrestling shoes, or Converse Chucks. Having your feet flat on the floor lessens the distance you have to pull the bar on a deadlift, increasing your leverage and helping you lift heavier weights. Training barefoot also strengthens your feet, which in turn adds stability and traction to all your lifts.

2.
BE A TIGHT-ASS

Squeeze your glutes at all times during a set, especially on lifts like the bench press and overhead press. It stabilizes your entire torso.

3.
USE THE 25-REP METHOD

If the total number of reps you perform for an exercise adds up to 25, you're more likely to maximize muscle and strength gains. Just keep the reps relatively low and the sets moderate. Configurations like 5x5, 6x4, and 8x3 work well.

4.
GO HEAVY, THEN LIGHT

Train with heavy loads one month, using sets of four to six reps. The next month, go lighter and stay in the 10–12 rep range. The heavy training allows your body to make even faster gains during the lighter weeks.

5.
THROW A MEDICINE BALL

Hold an 8- to 10-pounder and throw it hard into a wall a few feet in front of you, as if you were passing a basketball down the court. You can also reach overhead with the ball and then slam it hard into the floor. Do three sets of five reps. Explosive exercises fire up the central nervous system, helping you recruit more muscle fibers on lifts.

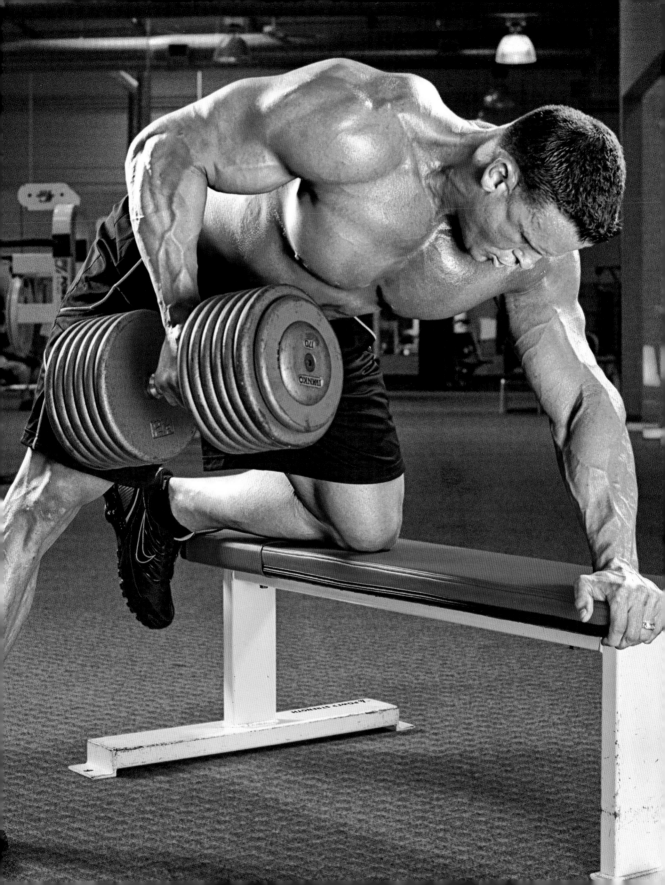

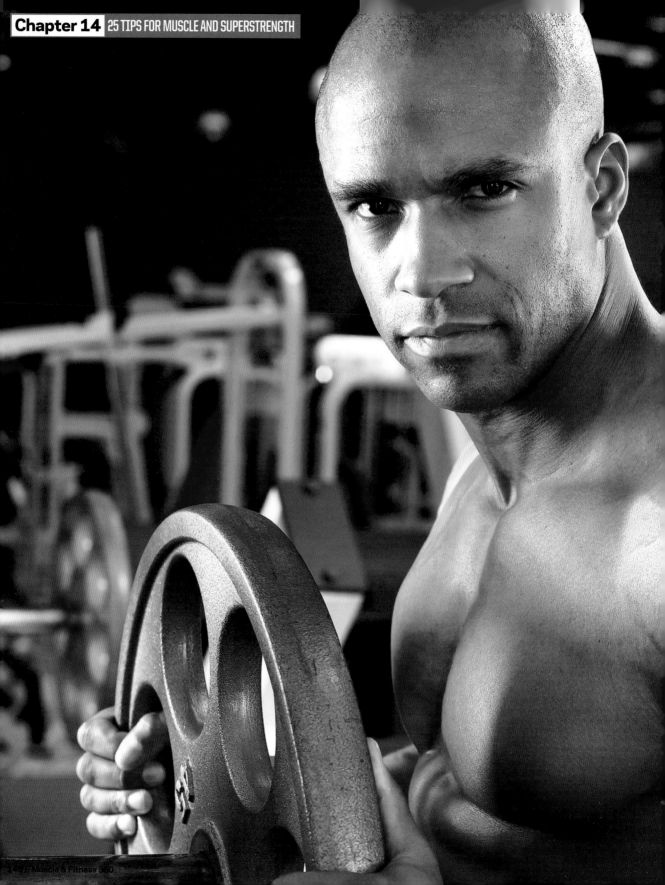

6.
TRAIN DELTS TO SHRINK YOUR WAIST

Want to look leaner without dieting? Develop the taper from your shoulders to your waist with this shoulder shocker: Hold a dumbbell in each hand. Now perform a lateral raise with your left arm. Keep your arm held up while you do a lateral raise with the right arm. Lower the right arm a quarter of the way down, raise it back up, then lower it all the way. Perform 10 reps like this. Rest three minutes, then switch arms. Perform one set first thing during your workout twice a week for four weeks.

7.
USE A NEUTRAL GRIP

If your sticking point on the bench press is at the bottom of the lift when the bar is on your chest, work on dumbbell bench presses with your palms facing each other. This positioning also forces you to tuck your elbows close to your sides when you lower the weights, which will become a habit when you press with a barbell. Benching with elbows tucked makes for a safer, stronger lift.

8.
MAKE YOUR WARMUP SET HEAVIER

Here's a great bait-and-switch trick for the nervous system. Work up in weight as normal on a lift to warm up, but make your last warm-up set a few pounds heavier than the load you plan to use for your first work set. Just make sure you per-form fewer reps in the warmup set than in the work set. So, if you want to squat 315 for five, you might work up to 320 or 325 in your last warmup set for two reps—it shouldn't be very difficult or tiring. Rest, then back off to 315 and go for five reps as planned. The set should feel easier than it would've otherwise, and you might try to go heavier next week.

9.
USE GRIP TOOLS

Wrap a towel around the bar or dumbbell handle to make the grip thicker—products like Grip4orce (*grip4orce.com*) and Fat Gripz (*fatgripz.com*) work even better. Increasing the challenge to your grip with any exercise recruits more muscles in your hands and forearms. As a result, you can bring up these areas fast without any extra isolation work.

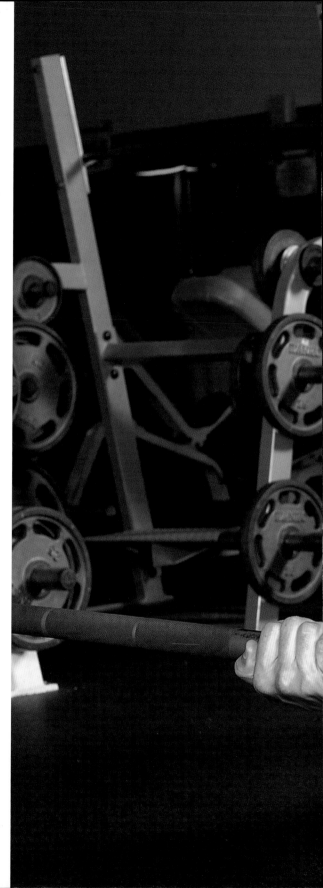

10.
DO PULLUPS TWICE A DAY

Do one set of as many as you can in the morning. Do another all-out set at night. Repeat this every other day. After 30 days, test your max number of reps. You can expect to see up to a 10-rep increase. This system works for dips as well.

11.
TAKE DIGESTIVE ENZYMES

If you're bulking up, taking in loads of extra food can be stressful to your gut and lead to poor absorption of nutrients. Digestive enzymes help break down that food. Make sure the ones you take contain protease, amylase, and lipase, which break down protein, starch, and fat, respectively.

12.
TRAIN ON EMPTY

The *European Journal of Applied Physiology* found that working out first thing in the morning on an empty stomach doubled the magnitude of muscle growth signals.

13.
DON'T LET YOUR ELBOWS MOVE WHEN CURLING

If you let them drift, you won't fully extend them, and you'll be cheating yourself out of a full range of motion.

14.
GO HEAVY

To build muscle, most of your sets need to be performed with weights that are at least 70% of your max weight for that exercise. This generally necessitates keeping reps to 12 and under.

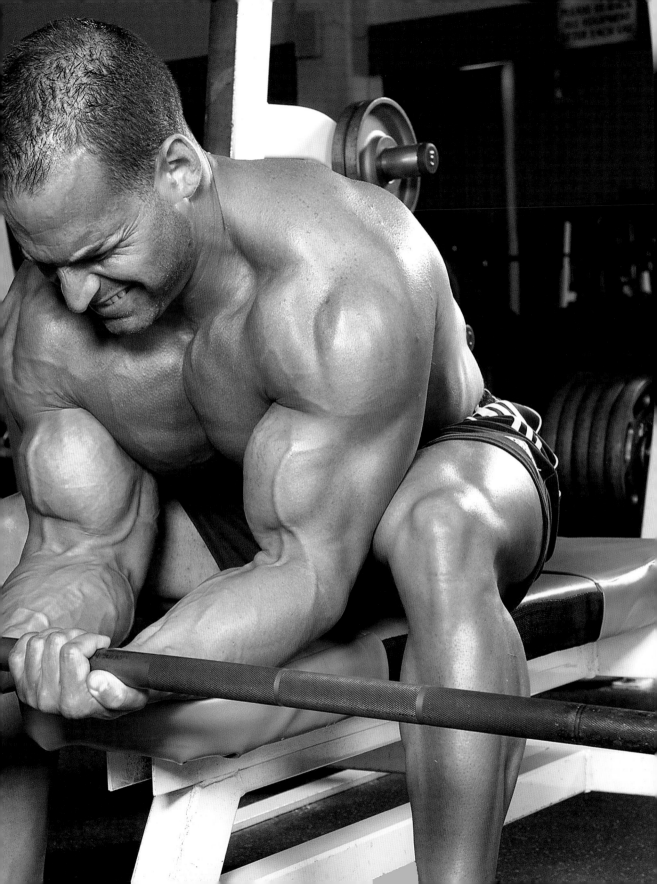

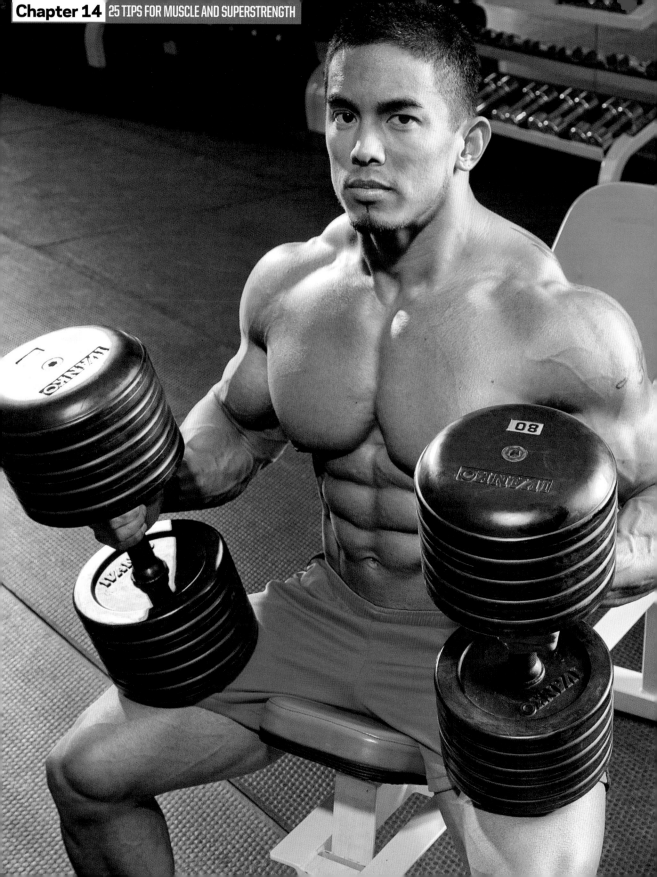

15.
DO "ISO HOLD" DROPSETS

Hold a weight in the contracted position (usually the top of the lift) and have a partner take off plates or reduce the load. It forces your muscles to keep working through the weight change. Unlike with regular dropsets in which the lifter will usually get a few seconds to recover, you get no rest doing this. This technique works well for machine exercises like Hammer Strength or Smith machine chest or shoulder presses. It's also great for barbell curls.

16.
TRY POST-EXHAUSTION

You may be familiar with "pre-exhaustion," in which you do an isolation exercise followed by a compound movement. This will tire out the bigger muscle groups you're training, forcing you to use less weight on the compound lift. However, the compound movement is the one that helps you make the quickest gains. Instead, try flipping it around, performing the compound move first, then repping out with the isolation. For example, do a set of bench presses and then pick up dumbbells for flyes.

17.
DRIVE YOUR TOES INTO THE FRONT OF YOUR SHOES

Coordinate this action with the upward phase of a bench press, right as you push the bar off your chest. The drive of your legs will actually allow you to handle more weight.

18.
USE PULLUP AIDS

If you can't do a pullup, lessening your body weight with the assistance of elastic bands makes the movement easier. Loop a thick exercise band around a pullup bar and place your feet in it. The band will act as a slingshot to propel you over the bar. The Pullup Revolution Pro (available at *lifelineusa.com*) offers various levels of assistance depending on your strength.

19.
USE THE TOTAL-REP METHOD

When you're looking to change things up, choose a weight you can get about 10 reps with, and aim for 30 total for that exercise. Perform each rep explosively and take as many sets as you need to get up to 30. The quality of your reps will likely be better, and you'll let your body determine the optimal number of sets.

20.
TRY CURLS ON LOWER-BODY DAYS

You'll be fresher than if you had just done back exercises and able to train the biceps more frequently. Now you'll be hitting them not just with legs, but indirectly on back day as well.

21.
FOLLOW LINEAR PERIODIZATION

Work up to a final set of eight reps on all your main barbell lifts for three weeks. Then go for a heavy five the next three weeks. Then three reps. Do just one hard work set per lift, then back it off by 10% and do another set of the same reps. Each wave builds on the gains of the previous one, and you should be setting personal records by the end of nine weeks.

22.
PUT YOUR BALL TO THE WALL

Before any big pressing workout, take a light medicine ball and press it into a wall with your arm extended. Roll the ball around and make the shape of all 26 letters. Keep pressure on the ball so it doesn't slip. This fires up the rotator cuff so you can stabilize heavy loads better.

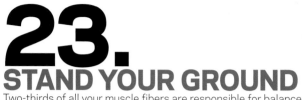

23.
STAND YOUR GROUND

Two-thirds of all your muscle fibers are responsible for balance and coordination. The remaining third are designed for movement. Therefore, you get more out of exercises that are done standing than you do ones where you're seated, lying down, or strapped into a machine.

24.
USE HYDROLYSATES IN YOUR POST-WORKOUT SHAKE

Proteins that have been "hydrolyzed" digest superfast, so your muscles soak them up quickly. The fast absorption also spikes levels of insulin. Try adding hydrolysates to your whey and carb post-workout shake to boost its efficacy.

25.
ROLL THE BAR UP TO YOUR SHINS TO DEADLIFT

Stand behind the bar, bend down to grab it, and then roll it back toward you. Just as it touches your shins, drop your butt and begin the lift. Time it right and you'll generate momentum that aids in the lift.

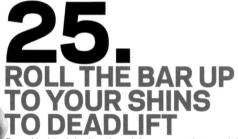

FAT-SEARING SEVEN

If a picture is worth a thousand words, then take a moment to conjure the physique of Maurice Greene, one of the greatest sprinters to have ever dug his spikes into the red rubber hide of a 400-meter oval. We featured him several years ago in *M&F* for one very good reason: He's got muscle—and not just in his legs. In fact, if there's one hallmark of the great sprinters of our time, it's their quarter horse-like physiques: densely muscled thighs propelling barrel-chested torsos down tracks at dangerously high speeds. The equivalent doesn't really exist on the long-distance side of the equation.

Envision a marathon runner and what do you come up with? A spindle-shanked Kenyan in short shorts. We first told you about HIIT, or high-intensity interval training, in *M&F* several years ago. Based on the latest research regarding interval training routines, HIIT tapped the well of exercise science to show conclusively that short, lung-searing bouts of cardio are more effective at burning fat than longer, steady-pace turns on the treadmill or exercise bike.

Among the chief benefits to test subjects was an increased resting metabolism over the subsequent 24 hours that resulted in a greater number of calories burned than their more languidly trained brethren. Although the overall calorie dump during exercise was higher for the steady-state subjects in one study's head-to-head comparisons, those on the HIIT program lost significantly more body fat—and that's the objective here.

Before we bore you into fat gain by documenting all the research in favor of sprint work, let us be clear: Science is on the side of HIIT as the most efficient way to burn fat while preserving muscle mass. But you don't really need science to tell you that; the empirical reality of the benefits of sprint work has been blowing down red rubber tracks before our eyes for years.

Just consider Greene and the Kenyan. Is there any question about whose physique you're after?

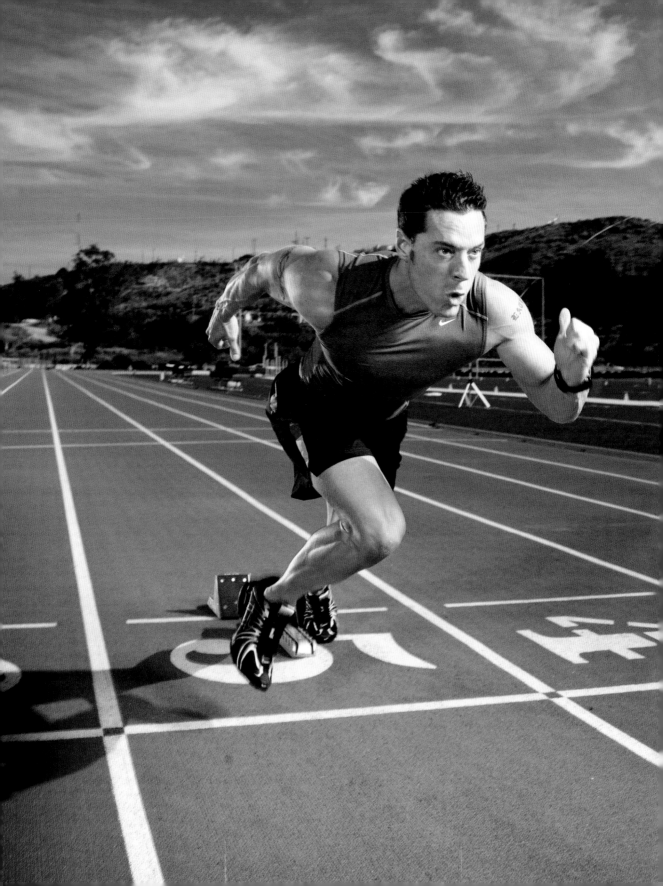

ON TR

We typically provide interval training programs designed for treadmills and exercise bikes, partly because most of you do your cardio in the gym and partly because track work in the biting cold of winter appeals only to Russo-Siberians in Murmansk.

But by taking your workouts to a local track when the weather allows, you're in effect periodizing your cardio to keep your body from acclimating to the same old routines, and you're countering the desire to drop your cardio altogether. The advantages of the seven sprint workouts presented here are variety, adaptability and ease of use. You don't need a heart-rate monitor or even a personal trainer to push buttons for you. You need a track, a watch and some good shoes.

Some people insist that steady, long-duration cardio (30–60 minutes) is the best way to get fit and lose fat, but we're here to tell you that shorter bouts of intense work can reap even bigger benefits for you. When faced with a small window in which to get your cardio done, you're better off speeding around a track a few times than strolling on a treadmill for an hour.

Depending on your goals, use our programs one to three times per week, not every day, and use just one of the interval options per day. Some are shorter than 30 minutes, some longer, so choose according to your schedule.

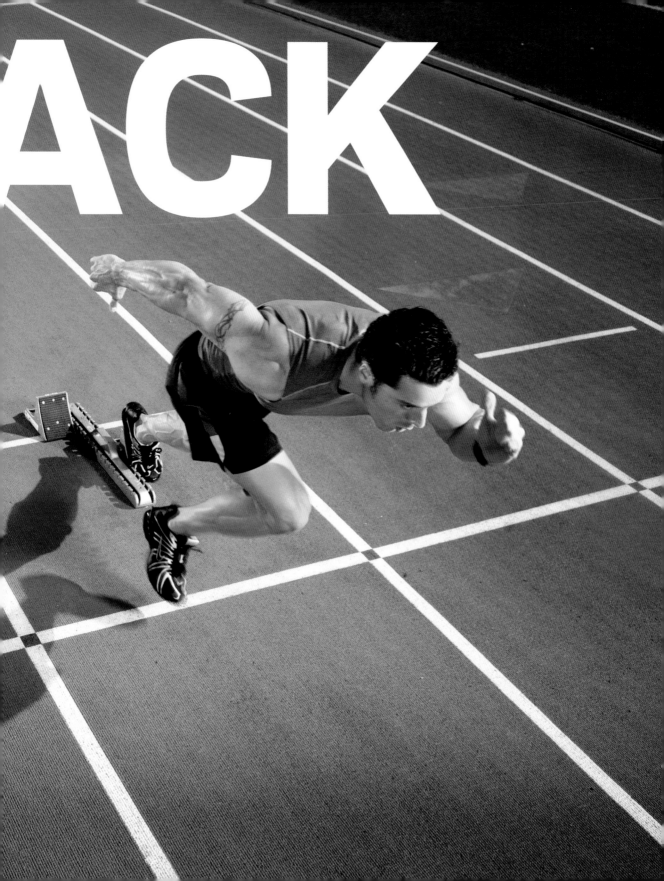

ACK

SPRINT W

Some of the sprint intervals in this article aren't for the faint of heart. But with seven options, there's something for everyone, and the variety will keep your workouts from becoming tedious before their time. Where you see "sprint-to-stride" (on the 30-second and one-minute sprint options), maintain your pace for as long as possible, then as you fatigue, slow down but keep pushing hard until the end.

Before each workout, take 5–10 minutes to warm up. Make sure you stretch appropriately so your muscles' range of motion is sufficient for the sprinting ahead. And for convenience's sake, do your best to find an actual track.

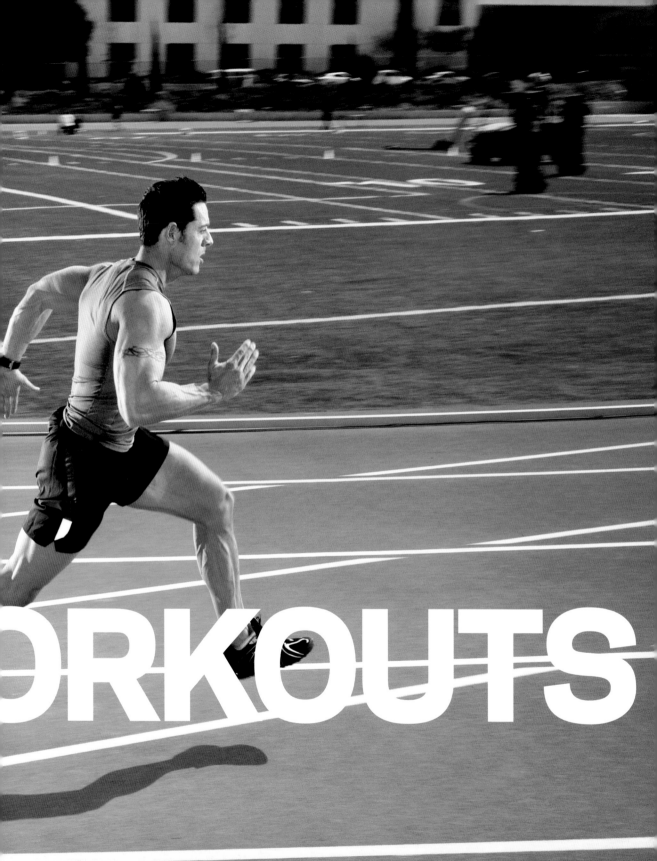

ORKOUTS

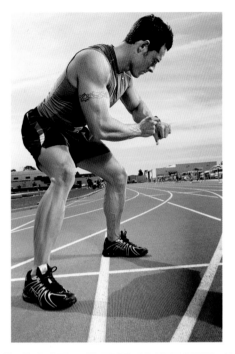

10-SECOND SPRINT TRAINING
TOTAL TIME 20 MINUTES

INTERVAL
10-SECOND SPRINT + ONE-MINUTE JOG

Repeat for a total of 20 minutes
This is a continuous-motion interval. Do not stop between sprints: Ease into the one-minute jogs, then ramp back up into the sprints.

BRIEF & BRUTAL SPRINT PROGRAM
TOTAL TIME 24–32 MINUTES

INTERVAL
30-SECOND SPRINT-TO-STRIDE + ONE-MINUTE WALK

Repeat three times
Walk for two minutes.
Repeat cycle two or three times.

THE MINUTE MAN
TOTAL TIME 32–48 MINUTES

INTERVAL
ONE-MINUTE SPRINT-TO-STRIDE + TWO-MINUTE WALK

Repeat three times
Walk for four minutes.
Repeat cycle one or two times.

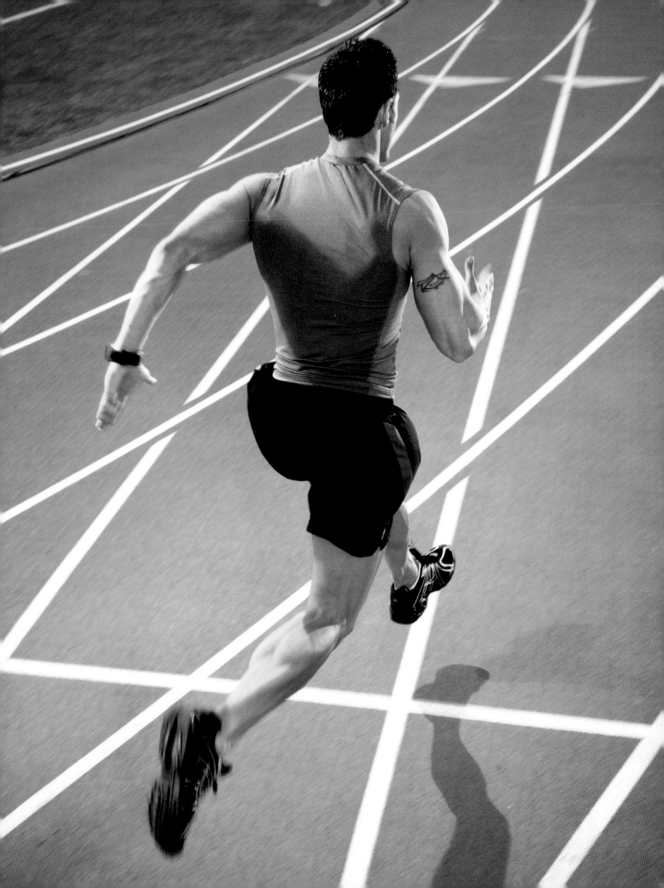

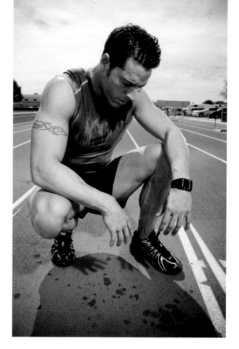

OUT OF THE BLOCKS
TOTAL TIME 25–30 MINUTES

INTERVAL
40-yard sprint + walk back to start.
Rest for two minutes after each sprint as you walk back to the start.
Complete 10 sprints total.

UP & BACK INTERVAL
TOTAL TIME 25–30 MINUTES

INTERVAL
Sprint 100 meters + walk back to start.
Sprint 200 meters + walk back to start.
Sprint 300 meters + walk back to start.
Sprint 400 meters + walk back to start.
Rest five minutes, then repeat cycle in reverse order.

4x4 INTERVAL
TOTAL TIME ABOUT 30 MINUTES

INTERVAL
100-meter sprint + walk 100 meters.
Repeat three times.
Rest for three minutes, then repeat two more times.

SEVEN THE HARD WAY
TOTAL TIME 25–35 MINUTES

INTERVAL
Seven 40-meter sprints + walk back to start.
Seven 100-meter sprints + walk back to start.
After each sprint, rest an additional 30 seconds beyond the time it takes
to walk back, then repeat.
If you're up for an additional challenge: Instead of 40- and 100-meter sprints,
do 100- and 200-meter sprints.

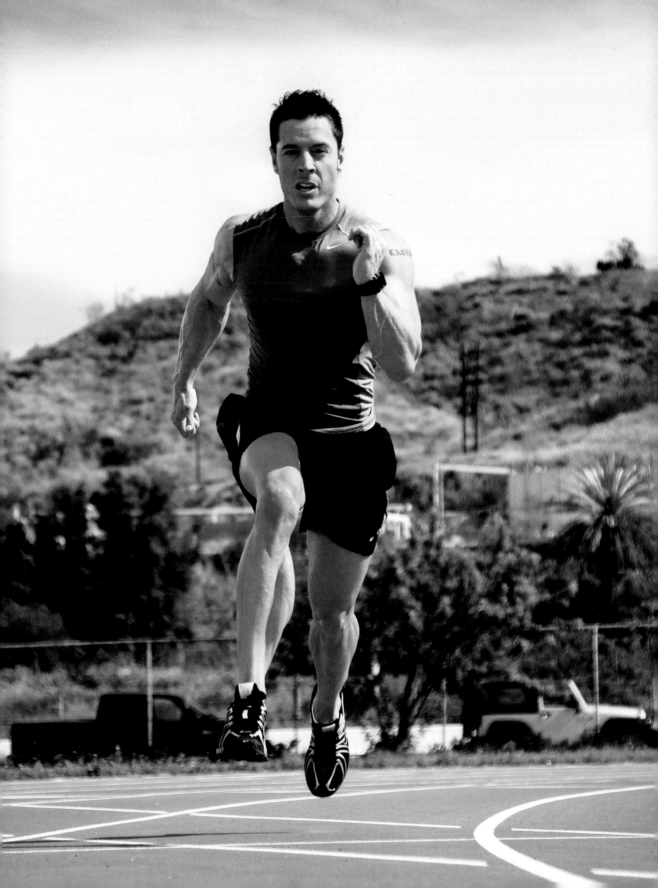

21 FOODS YOU SHOULD NEVER BE WITHOUT

Eating the right foods to feed your muscles and fuel your physical endeavors can be compared to an expert-level Sudoku puzzle: confusing and frustrating, and you don't want to meet the guy who's good at it. In reality, designing a meal plan that'll help you achieve your fitness goals is as simple as buying these 21 foods and constantly replenishing them. These choices are heavy on antioxidants, fiber, healthy fats, protein, and slow-burning carbs; and light on chemicals, empty calories, sugar, and trans fats. Bottom line: If you were stuck on a desert island with these foods and a barbell, you'd hit all your training goals.

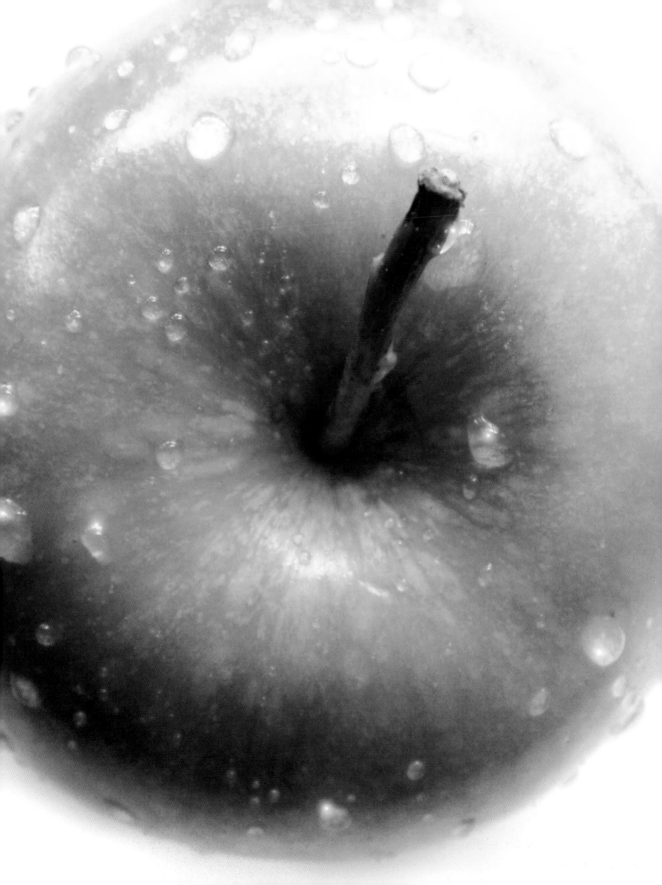

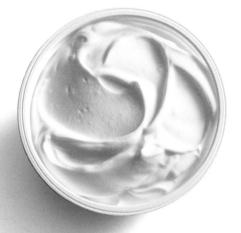

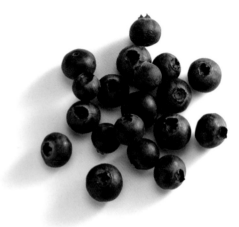

1.
GREEK YOGURT

This stuff has a wealth of gut-friendly probiotic bacteria and calcium, which helps burn fat, and it contains almost twice the protein of regular yogurt. A caveat: Check the sugar content, as some Greek yogurts can be overloaded with the sweet stuff. Plain is always best.

> *8 oz of 2%: 150 calories, 20g protein, 6g carbs, 4g fat, 3g sat fat, 0g fiber*

2.
BEANS

Besides being ridiculously cheap, beans are one of nature's nutritional all-stars. They deliver a monster dose of fat-obliterating fiber plus folate, iron, magnesium, zinc (which raises testosterone levels), and a healthy amount of protein. Add your favorite variety to chili, salad, and soup.

> *1 cup black beans: 227 calories, 15g protein, 41g carbs, 1g fat, 0g sat fat, 15g fiber*

3.
BLUEBERRIES

The blueberry's ascension to nutritional sainthood is well-deserv[...] Research reports that its potent antioxidant anthocyanin helps b[...] ish belly fat and shields the brain from oxidative damage. Add wi[...] blueberries wherever you can for the biggest antioxidant punch.

> *1 cup: 84 calories, 1g protein, 21g carbs, 0g fat, 0g sat fat, 4g fiber*

4.
BROCCOLI

This nutritional overachiever is chock-full of fat-busting fiber, folate, and vitamins C and K. Broccoli also contains the antioxida[...] sulforaphane, which helps fight cancer. This cruciferous vegetab[...] may reduce excess estrogen levels in the body and, in turn, prevent fat storage.

> *1 cup: 31 calories, 3g protein, 6g carbs, 0g fat, 0g sat fat, 2g fiber*

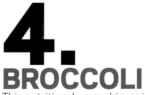
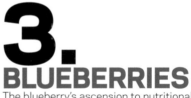

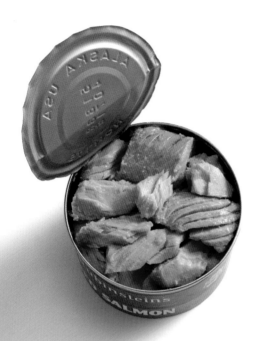

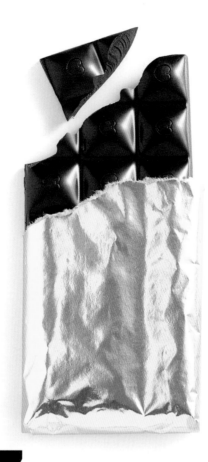

5.
CANNED SALMON

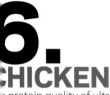

...cked with protein and exceptionally convenient, canned ...mon is a better source of calcium, omega-3 fatty acids ...d vitamin D than tuna. Research suggests the healthy fats ...t belly bulge by improving insulin sensitivity and reducing ...storage while ramping up fat oxidation. Use canned salmon ...andwiches and mix into salads.

...oz pink salmon: 152 calories, 24g protein, 0g carbs, ...fat, 1g sat fat, 0g fiber

6.
CHICKEN

...protein quality of ultraversatile chicken ranks up there with ...er heavyweights such as beef, eggs, and fish because it's easily ...thesized to repair muscle tissue and help it grow. As a bonus, ...ultry is rich in niacin, a B vitamin essential for the conversion of ...bohydrates, fat, and protein into usable energy.

...oz breast meat: 186 calories, 36g protein, ...carbs, 2g fat, 1g sat fat, 0g fiber

7.
DARK CHOCOLATE

A small amount of dietary cheating can prevent a fast and furious slide into gluttony. Dark chocolate is as good a cheat food as you can find because of its polyphenol antioxidants, which reduce the risk of heart disease and stroke. Chocolate is calorically dense, so limit yourself to 1–2 ounces a day, and make sure your bar of choice contains at least 60% cocoa for more polyphenols and less sugar.

> 1 oz: 162 calories, 2g protein, 15g carbs, 11g fat, 6g sat fat, 2g fiber

8.
EGGS

Think of eggs—yolk and all—as a bodybuilding MVP that delivers vital nutrients such as vitamins A, B12, and D, selenium, and easily absorbed protein in just a few calories. The protein in eggs may reduce blood pressure and protect against cardiovascular disease, according to Canadian research published in 2009. What's more, eating eggs at breakfast can satisfy your hunger and prevent overeating later.

> 1 large egg: 71 calories, 6g protein, 0g carbs, 5g fat, 2g sat fat, 0g fiber

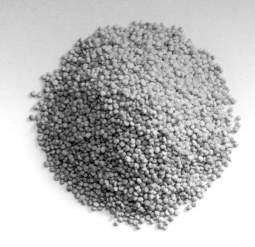

9.
GRASS-FED BEEF

This protein-packed treat possesses more fat-busting conjugated linoleic acid, anti-inflammatory omega-3 fatty acids, and vitamin E than its corn-fed brethren. Plus, it tastes like beef should. Look for the words "loin" and "round," which are the leanest cuts. Bison is another stellar red-meat pick.

> **6 oz tenderloin: 258 calories, 36g protein, 0g carbs, 12g fat, 6g sat fat, 0g fiber**

10.
QUINOA

This whole-grain powerfood of the Incas contains muscle-building essential amino acids—very rare among grains—and plenty of fiber; iron; and magnesium, an often-underconsumed mineral that helps control blood-sugar levels. Plus, quinoa cooks twice as fast as brown rice.

> **1 cup: 222 calories, 8g protein, 39g carbs, 4g fat, 0g sat fat, 5g fiber**

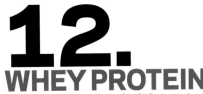

11.
SHRIMP

These crustaceans possess an unbeatable protein-to-fat ratio, plus they're an excellent source of the antioxidant selenium and are one of the few food sources of vitamin D, a vital nutrient in which many active guys are deficient. Keep a bag of precooked frozen shrimp on hand to thaw and toss into pasta, salad, and soup.

> 16 large shrimp: 120 calories, 24g protein, 0g carbs, 1g fat, 0g sat fat, 0g fiber

12.
WHEY PROTEIN

The fast-digesting branched-chain amino acids in whey are just what a body needs after a tough workout to build shirt-stretching muscle. Research from the University of Connecticut (Storrs) shows that the protein peptides in whey can stimulate blood flow, which could increase nutrient delivery to muscles and improve heart health.

> 1 scoop vanilla: 120 calories, 23g protein, 2g carbs, 2g fat, 1g sat fat, 0g fiber

13.
RED BELL PEPPER

In the vegetable world, red bell peppers are the vitamin C heavy-weight champ. Besides acting as a powerful antioxidant, vitamin C helps produce carnitine, a compound required for fat oxidation. Bell peppers also contain lycopene, an antioxidant that protects against prostate cancer. Roasted (jarred) red bell peppers are just as nutritious as fresh.

> *1 cup: 46 calories, 1g protein, 9g carbs, 0g fat, 0g sat fat, 3g fiber*

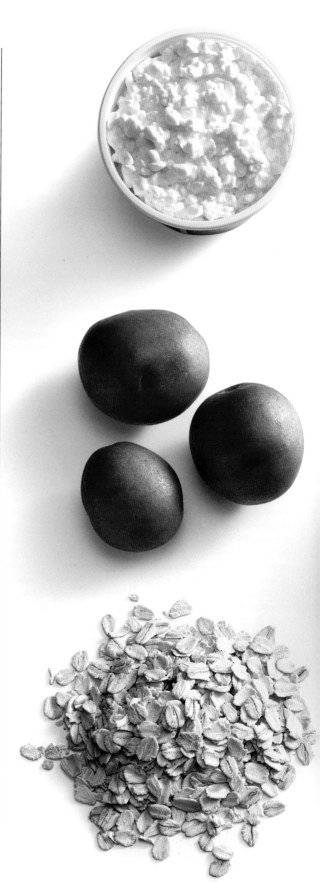

14.
LOW-FAT COTTAGE CHEESE

The protein in cottage cheese is predominantly casein, which is slow-digesting and provides muscles with a steady supply of amino acids. This makes cottage cheese ideal before bed to minimize catabolism during the night. To keep fat calories in line, opt for 1% milk fat.

> *1 cup: 163 calories, 28g protein, 6g carbs, 2g fat, 1g sat fat, 0g fiber*

15.
POTATOES

Despite what you hear, white potatoes aren't just a source of belt-expanding calories. Post-workout, nosh on one to spike levels of the anabolic hormone insulin, which drives amino acids, carbs, and creatine into muscle cells to replace spent energy stores; and to stimulate muscle repair and growth. Spuds also harbor fat-busting fiber; blood pressure-lowering potassium; iron for energy; and vitamin C, which helps encourage muscle recovery.

> *1 large potato: 278 calories, 7g protein, 63g carbs, 0g fat, 0g sat fat, 7g fiber*

16.
PLAIN OATS

This slow-digesting breakfast favorite promotes fat-burning during exercise and squashes cravings. What's more, it contains the soluble fiber beta-glucan, which keeps blood-sugar and cholesterol levels in check. If you have ample time, opt for less-processed steel-cut oats, which digest even slower and have more antioxidants and fiber.

> *1/2 cup dry: 154 calories, 6g protein, 28g carbs, 3g fat, 1g sat fat, 4g fiber*

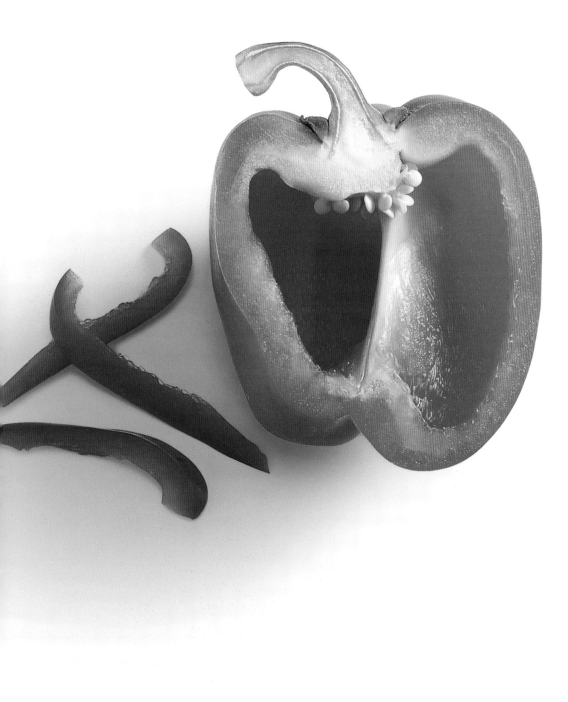

17.
SPROUTED BREAD

Made from sprouted whole grains and legumes, sprouted bread has more protein than any other. The sprouting process also pumps up the dietary fiber, minerals, and vitamins, and gives it a nutty flavor. Furthermore, each slice is lower than other breads on the glycemic index, a measure of how fast a food spikes blood sugar. This reduces the potential for fat storage and provides a steadier supply of energy to power you through the day.

> *2 slices: 160 calories, 10g protein, 28g carbs, 1g fat, 0g sat fat, 6g fiber*

18.
SPINACH

This leafy green veggie contains beta-ecdysterone, a phytochemical that has anabolic properties. Spinach is also crammed with immune-boosting vitamins A and K, which strengthens bones.

> *2 cups raw: 14 calories, 2g protein, 2g carbs, 0g fat, 0g sat fat, 2g fiber*

19.
APPLES

Quercetin, the flavonoid antioxidant found in apples, has anti-inflammatory properties that can improve exercise endurance and health. Researchers from the University of South Carolina (Columbia) found that quercetin may protect those who exercise hard from the flu by boosting their immune systems.

> *1 medium apple: 95 calories, 0g protein, 25g carbs, 0g fat, 0g sat fat, 4g fiber*

20.
EXTRA-VIRGIN OLIVE OIL

Olive oil is rich in heart-healthy monounsaturated fat as well as oleocanthal, a polyphenol compound that behaves like a natural anti-inflammatory to help soothe gym-worn muscles. Australian scientists found that heat reduces oleocanthal's effectiveness, so keep extra-virgin olive oil out of the sauté pan; instead, use it on salad and potatoes.

> *1 tbsp: 119 calories, 0g protein, 0g carbs, 14g fat, 2g sat fat, 0g fiber*

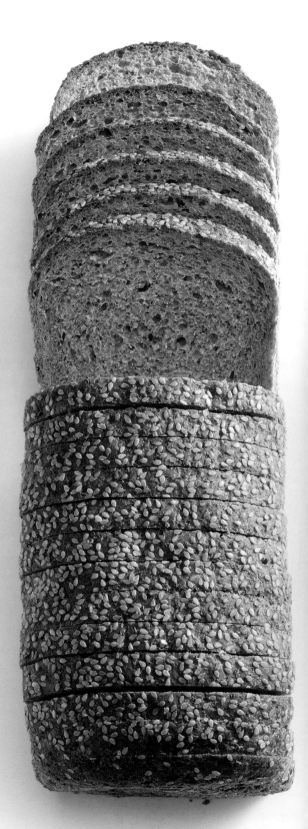

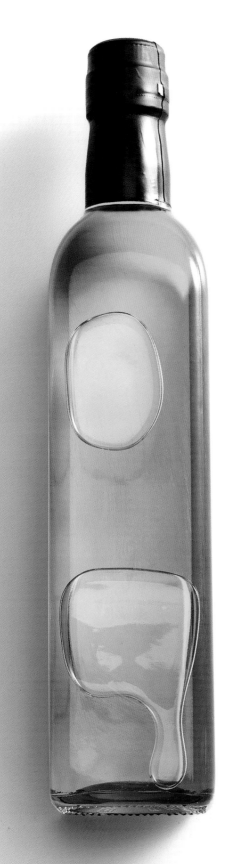

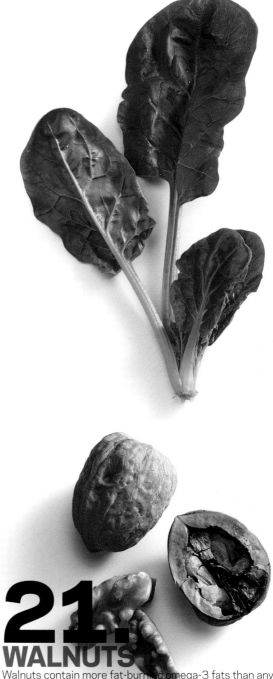

21.
WALNUTS

Walnuts contain more fat-burning omega-3 fats than any other nut, and research continues to show that those who eat them regularly more easily win the war on flab. Harvard University scientists recently found that diets rich in walnuts could slash cholesterol levels. They can be frozen and stored for long periods.
> *1 oz: 185 calories, 4g protein, 4g carbs, 18g fat, 2g sat fat, 2g fiber*